Stop Binge Eating 101

How To Overcome Compulsive and Emotional Eating

Monica E. Harris

Disclaimer: The content in this book, Stop Binge Eating 101, is not intended to be a substitute for professional medical advice, diagnosis, or treatment. Always seek the advice of your physician or other qualified health provider with any questions you may have regarding a medical condition. Never disregard professional medical advice or delay in seeking it because of something you have read in this book. Reliance on any information found in this book is solely at your own risk.

The author and publisher assume no responsibility for any outcome of the use of this book in self-treatment or under the care of a licensed doctor or physician.

While every precaution has been taken in the preparation of this book, the publisher assumes no responsibility for errors or omissions, or for damages resulting from the use of the information contained herein.

This book is for entertainment and informational purposes only. The views expressed are those of the author alone and should not be taken as expert instruction or commands. The reader is responsible for his or her own actions. Neither the author nor the publisher assumes any responsibility or liability whatsoever on behalf of the purchaser or reader of these materials. The reader is responsible for their own use of any products or methods mentioned in this publication.

This book includes information about products and equipment offered by third parties. As such, the author does not assume responsibility or liability for any third party products or opinions. Third party product manufacturers have not sanctioned this book, nor does the author receive any compensation from said manufacturers for sharing information regarding their products.

Stop Binge Eating 101
First edition. July 1, 2020.
Copyright © 2020 Monica E. Harris

Table of Contents

Introduction

I didn't want to stop overeating.

There. I said it.

Ice cream, pizza, potato chips, chocolate, any fried food... the list goes on and on. My favorite foods bring me a sense of comfort and, yes, sometimes, even joy. The actual problem is that I don't want to enjoy these foods in moderation. I want to keep eating until I can't eat anymore... and then I want to eat some more.

I have felt the shame of eating twice as much as everyone else at the dinner table. I've made promises to myself about dieting that have been broken as quickly as I could consume a box of double chocolate chip cookies. I've felt judgment from friends and family that criticize my eating choices. Many times, not because they want to hurt me, but rather because they love me.

This unhealthy habit is a real problem. Not only does it impact my health, but it hinders me from living my best life.

Maybe you can relate. And now that you understand a little about my struggle, you know you're not alone.

For me, something had to change. I couldn't see a future where life was different, but I knew I couldn't continue down this road. Not only did I change my life, but I am passionate about helping others overcome binge eating.

Overeating is not as uncommon as you may think. Research has shown that Binge Eating Disorder (BED) is treated in four out of ten individuals who are trying to lose weight.

So, are you struggling with binge eating or overeating?

6

Take a look at these signs and symptoms:

- You eat when you aren't hungry.
- You eat when you're full.
- Your eating habits feel out of control.
- You eat unusually large portions of food in a short amount of time.
- You feel embarrassed, guilty, or disgusted by your eating habits.
- You eat in secret or hide food that can be eaten at another time.
- You are continually dieting with no positive results.

If you identified with one or more of those statements, you are most likely somewhere on the overeating spectrum.

The good news is that this pattern can be broken and you can establish new habits that will enable you to begin living the life you've always wanted. You don't have to wait for something magical to happen that forces you to stop binge eating. It starts by simply choosing to change how you view food.

Now, before you stop reading because I've made changing your entire lifestyle sound far too easy, just wait. I don't want to trivialize how difficult it is to stop overeating. In fact, part of that choice may include reaching out for medical or psychological help, but self-help is a great place to start.

Having will power is not enough to fight off cravings that are so strong that they interrupt everything in your daily life. I realize that this change may result in emptying your pantry and refrigerator and making a clean start. But it's worth it to become a healthier version of yourself – you are worth it.

In the following pages, we will take a journey together. We will get to the root of when and how overeating became a part of your life. Then, we will explore how you can develop a new, healthy view of food. It won't happen overnight, and it won't be easy, but it's worth the sacrifice to live healthier and extend the length of your life.

In our present culture, overeating has often been trivialized as a lapse in judgment or poor lifestyle choices that result in eating too much. However, this disorder crosses gender and societal boundaries and has proven to be a much deeper issue. Those who struggle with perfectionism, high levels of anxiety, and social pressures find themselves at risk.

In 2003, the American Psychiatric Association (APA) recognized Binge Eating Disorder (BED) as a psychiatric disorder. This gave way for diagnosis and treatment for those who are suffering in a way like never before. It legitimized the seriousness of this disorder and those who suffer from it.

According to the National Institute of Health (NIH), Binge Eating Disorder (BED) is the most prevalent eating disorder, more common than anorexia and bulimia combined.

The Eating Disorder Foundation notes that BED is similar to anorexia and bulimia in how an individual needs to be in control. This is a constant internal struggle for those who overeat. When they binge eat, they recognize that once again, they have lost control. This can result in low self-esteem, depression, feelings of defeat and disgust, and distress. Some people are even impaired and crippled to the point they can't function in their everyday life.

However, when you learn to manage overeating, you begin the process of coping with your emotions, thoughts, and struggles with food.

So, if you are struggling with overeating, I promise that you will be in a better place by the end of this book. You will be equipped with tools that enable you to control what you eat and where food no longer controls you.

Today is the day you can choose to travel down a different path. You *can* establish new eating habits, and you *can* change the entire course of your life. However, if you decide to remain in the place you are right now, your overall mental and physical health will be at risk.

Those who struggle with binge eating often have problems at work, they avoid being around others, and generally have a poor quality of life. Typically, their physical complications include a laundry list of medical conditions such as heart disease, diabetes, joint problems, and more.

This book will offer helpful advice from leading eating disorder authorities. I will share my own story and what steps I have personally taken to become healthy. I'm a different person than I used to be. I've grown from painful experiences and have found healing in my mind and body as I've taken time to process the new me.

I believe you can also discover your path to a healthier and happier lifestyle. In the next chapter, we'll take the first step on this journey together.

Chapter 1: Identify the Root of Overeating

What Is Binge Eating/Overeating?

Overeating Versus Binge Eating

While many people use the terms synonymously, overeating and binge eating are not the same. There's a good deal of overlap in these ideas, and overeating *is* one component of binge eating, but those who overeat are *not necessarily* binge eaters. Moreover, binge eaters inevitably experience overeating. Overeating is a part of life, while binge eating is a serious and often debilitating condition. Know the differences between these two concepts to better understand your relationship with food and judge if your problem has risen to the level of binge eating. If it hasn't, you still need to be aware that overeating can quickly spiral into binge eating, so whoever you are, you need to ensure that you have a healthy relationship with food and that what you eat doesn't control how happy you are or take up hours of mental exertion. Too many people spend way too much energy thinking about what they're eating.

Overeating is a normal experience that all people face at one point or another. If you have bouts of overeating, be vigilant, but don't worry too much because part of enjoying food means overindulging occasionally. These episodes of overeating shouldn't give you feelings of immense guilt. If you've ever eaten cake at a birthday party even though you weren't hungry, that could be classified as overeating. When you stuff yourself full of food on holidays, that is also overeating, but in these cases, the frequency of overeating is low, and in healthy overeating scenarios, you don't beat yourself up over your actions. You're able to move on without letting that occasion warp how you behave in future food encounters. You go about your life without feeling self-hate and dread at your overeating.

Binge eating, meanwhile, includes overeating, but binge eating takes overeating to a whole new level and puts your head in an unhealthy space. You often subscribe to black and white thinking, and your actions become cyclical. Binge eating comes with feelings of distress as well as physical discomfort. When you binge, you feel ashamed and out of control. Plus, for binging, the rate in which you eat food is generally more rapid than normal. You don't enjoy the food. You are hurriedly eating it and trying to get as much into your body as quickly as possible. You may feel like an awful person for doing this, even though how you eat has nothing to do with your worth as a person.

If you noticed that your overeating has become more frequent and more compulsive, you might be wandering into binge eating territory. If your episodes of binge eating are happening at a high frequency, you may qualify for a full-blown Binge Eating disorder diagnosis.

Binge Eating Disorder

This is an eating disorder that is marked by eating enormous quantities of food in brief periods of time, leading to guilt, shame, bloating, fullness, and a feeling of losing your autonomy over food. For short, this disorder is known as BED. For a diagnosis, patients must have binge eating episodes for three months at a rate of at least one binge per week; however, even if you don't meet this standard, an eating disorder may be developing so don't take your binge eating lightly no matter how frequently you engage in behaviors. If you're binging only twice a month, that's still too many, and the information in this book can help you free yourself from food worry for good.

Out of all eating disorders, BED is the most common; it impacts three percent of women as well as two percent of men at any given time. Eight percent of people will have suffered this disorder within their lifetime. Further, it is the eating disorder that is frequently triggered by pregnancy and hormonal changes that are often normal parts of life. Whereas the onset of eating disorders often occurs in adolescence or young adulthood, binge eating can more often have onsets later in life and impacts both men and women.

While it is one of the most prevalent eating disorders, it often doesn't get the same attention that other eating disorders like anorexia nervosa or bulimia nervosa receive. It has only recently been included as its own diagnosis in the DSM-V, which is the guide psychological experts use to diagnosis patients with psychological disorders. Before 2013, BED was categorized under the now eliminated category of Eating Disorder Not Otherwise Specified (EDNOS), which was a grouping of disorders that didn't fall under the more specifically defined eating disorder categories. Luckily, with increased attention, BED finally got its own category in the DSM, but there's still ongoing work researchers need to do to understand more about this disorder.

Some common symptoms of binge eating disorder are as follows:

1. Fast-paced eating.
2. Consuming large quantities of food in a single sitting.
3. Being unable to control your eating.
4. Feeling stuffed to the point of discomfort.
5. Eating even when you aren't hungry.
6. Isolating yourself when you eat.
7. Being disgusted with yourself for your actions, or feeling anxious and depressed by those actions.

Binge eating disorder does not include compensatory behaviors such as purging. Using purging behaviors such as vomiting, laxatives, compulsive exercise, or fasting to alleviate the anxiety of binging fall under the category of bulimia nervosa.

Some side effects that you may have because of binging include other mental health disorders such as anxiety or depression, diseases like diabetes or heart disease; insomnia; joint pain; and menstrual irregularities. Binging wreaks havoc on your body and causes your hormones and regular functioning of your body to be erratic. Even your skin and hair may suffer from binging. Plus, one of the worst areas that binging influences is your digestive system. Binging may result in increased heartburn and acid reflux, IBS, diarrhea, constipation, and stomach pain. In some cases, one's stomach may even rupture from being so full, so the dangers of binging are very real, and you must take them seriously.

Unfortunately, while data says that nearly ten million Americans suffer from this disorder currently, BED is widely underdiagnosed, and many people who have it never seek treatment. Often, shame and stigma lead to people not wanting to come forward with their struggles, making it a disorder that has been under-researched and is shrouded with secrecy, but with some education and helpful tips, you can put an end to your binge eating forever. It may seem impossible to cut it out of your life, but people do get better, myself included.

How to Identify if Binging Is a Problem?

If you're reading this book, you probably already suspect that you or someone you love may have a problem with binge eating. Chances are that even if you do not binge frequently enough for a BED diagnosis, you may have a binge eating problem. The fact that you are concerned about your eating habits shows that you probably have that out of control feeling when it comes to food. Even if you just overeat, the advice in this book can show you how to keep a healthy relationship with food and ensure that your bad habits don't lead to you developing an eating disorder.

Even though you've picked up this book, you might be saying to yourself, "I don't think my problems are bad enough to be serious, but I want them to stop," and that's a common mentality to have. Many people think that their issues aren't severe enough to be serious or that they're making a big deal out of nothing. On the contrary, eating disorders and disordered eating are always serious.

Being that humans must eat, you cannot escape food. Thus, if your relationship with eating is dysfunctional, you'll never be able to experience the joy and peace of mind that you deserve.

For a long time, I didn't realize that my food behaviors were a problem because of biases I wrongly held and the teachings of a weight-loss driven society. I thought that my binges were a result of a lack of will power and didn't understand why I couldn't get my act together and get the extra pounds off. I have since learned that my behavior was perfectly logical. It wasn't healthy, but there was a name for what I was experiencing, and being able to use the word binge after having no language for what I was doing helped me change my life and kick binge eating aside for good. It's been nearly seven years since I've last had a binge when at one point, I couldn't even go three days without one!

The first step is acknowledging that your relationship with food is warped. Don't try to belittle your problems because food should never be the enemy. It keeps you alive and gives you the power to do amazing things. Without food, you would die, so it's time to stop feeling bad for eating. Even if you eat too much, that's better than not eating enough to sustain your body as long as you've accepted that you can't control your urges and need to coexist with them.

If you have had multiple experiences of ingesting food far past the point of being full and feeling out of control around food, you likely have some kind of eating disorder or, at the very least disordered eating. If you find yourself constantly thinking about your next meal or worrying that you'll lose control at a buffet, you have a problem. Whenever food starts to take up hours of your time each day, that's when you know you need to change. Eating should be instinctual and feel good. You shouldn't be stressing out over every meal. If you are, yet again, that's an indicator of a problem. Trust your gut on this. If it is telling you that something is wrong, something probably is! Let yourself accept the help that you need. Most importantly, know that you're not going through this journey alone.

You're Not Alone

I began binge eating in junior high, maybe even younger, but my issues worsened when I was eighteen in my second semester in college, feeling like the worst person alive. I'd always been an emotional eater, eating to cope with whatever I was feeling, ranging from anxiety to sadness to joy. I used food as both a reward and punishment, and in the process, my relationship with eating became twisted. I began to dread food, even though it was the part of my day I most looked forward to. I began hiding out in my room and munching on all the chips and sweets I could find. I'd gorge myself on anything just to fill the pit in my stomach that constantly seemed to be begging for salt and sugar.

I was an active child, so for a while, I was able to engage in these behaviors without gaining weight. I still felt guilty for what I was doing, but in high school, I began putting on weight at a rapid pace, and I started feeling increasingly worse about myself. The lower my self-esteem dropped, the harder it became to control what I was eating, so I kept putting on weight, which made me feel more unhappy and led to more binge eating to cope with the self-hate I felt! My self-hate was about more than my weight, but at the time, I thought that losing weight would make everything better. When I got to college, I was so dissatisfied with myself that I was desperate to make changes as quickly as possible, and this want led to me abusing my body and confusing it.

My final downward spiral started with a very simple pursuit that I'd seen friends and family members experience for years: a diet. Wanting to counteract the freshman fifteen, I vowed to lose weight, and I didn't realize all the negative impacts that weight loss could have on my mind and body. When I started binging more frequently despite my dieting efforts, I felt out of control— like a monster— and I had no idea how to make it better, so I lived with the shame and guilt that come with binging, and I didn't think that anything would ever change. By day I tried to lose weight, but by night, I became the ravenous binge monster. I isolated myself from my friends and spent my spare time being hungry no matter how much I'd already eaten. I was in a war with my hunger, and I wasted countless hours fighting with myself to try to find a semblance of control over my body, which kept doing things that I didn't want it to do.

I spent over a decade battling my hunger, and I never felt so hopeless as I did then. During my extreme binging years, I felt that my binge eating made me a freak and separated me from my peers. I self-isolated and became ashamed of my behaviors rather than reaching out and seeking change. My entire lifestyle suffered because of my twisted relationship with food. Yet, even in the height of immense dysfunction, it took me a long time to want to change. To change, I had to realize how common binge eating is and how our culture encourages this problem more than it tries to prevent it. I had to learn that my disorder wasn't because I was a bad person; it was because of my circumstances as well as a society that failed me. While eating disorders have biological roots, they also have deep societal roots. Thus, you are not alone with your binge eating, and you shouldn't feel like your binge eating reflects poorly on your character because it is a common problem that is created by a culture that fixates on unsustainable methods of weight loss.

Who Is Impacted by Binge Eating?

Binge eating impacts a wide range of people, so anyone can have it. People of all genders, races, and socioeconomic classes face this issue. Further, binge eating can occur among people of any size. It is most common for binge eating to occur in obese people. Those with a family history of binge eating will be more likely to binge eat, and childhood trauma can increase people's chances of developing BED. It is more common, but not significantly, among women than men. Among women, binge eating begins between the ages of eighteen and twenty-nine while among men, this disorder is often seen later in life between the ages of forty-five and fifty-nine.

As for socioeconomic factors, research has suggested that binge eating may be more dependent on income for women than for men, but cases were also seen across social classes. A Project Eat experiment suggested that those of higher socioeconomic status were more prone to binge eating when they were dissatisfied with their bodies, dieted, and were mocked about their weight by family members. These factors, however, were not as influential on people of lower socioeconomic status. For those of lower socioeconomic status, factors like being obese or overweight, dieting, and not having good access to food often led to binge eating.

Whatever your circumstances, you may be at risk for binge eating disorder if you have any signs of frequent emotional eating or an otherwise warped relationship with food. Likewise, if you have an obsession with your weight or diet, you may also develop a problem with binging. While a range of factors leads to binge eating such as food scarcity and access to addictive, less nutritious foods, one of the biggest contributors to binge eating is a diet culture that promises fast, easy weight loss results.

The Culture of Binging and Why Dieting Is Bad

Unfortunately, we live in a culture that is fixated on the number on the scale more than it is fixated on the health of people who are pushed into unneccessary diets. Perfectly healthy people start diets every day just because it seems like they should. A social emphasis is put on weight, and in the process, people become predisposed to dieting, which often leads to binge eating because of the unrealistic parameters that diets have. Therefore, to fix your binge eating problem, you need to understand how diet culture plays into your issues and how to resist the allure of diets. Contrary to what you may think, you cannot stop binge eating if you continue to diet. Once you stop binging, you will be able to make healthier choices and eat more foods that nourish you on your journey to freedom from binging. For now, don't restrict yourself at all. To stop binge eating, you must vow to never go on a diet again. It may seem hard to promise this because the idea that you may never lose weight is painful to countless people, but I was at my heaviest weight when I was at the height of my binge eating due to the neverending hunger that filled me. I did eventually lose weight, but as I stopped dieting, I noticed I didn't worry about it as much. I was happy in my skin after years of hating who I was.

For a long time, I thought that if I could just find the right diet then I could lose weight and start eating normally. But the more I tried to resist my need for food, the more I binged, and the more weight I gained. It was an endless cycle of trying to deprive myself, getting fed up, binging, and feeling shame. I discovered that you can't force your body to be a size it doesn't want to be. So don't dream of being the weight of a model on the cover of a magazine. First of all, she's probably been heavily photoshopped, but more importantly, one size does not fit all. What's healthy for one person may not be healthy for you. People have natural body weights based on factors like genetics, so you shouldn't compare yourself to others to determine your health.

Some theorists have come up with the idea of a set point weight that all people have, which is a weight that your body tends to maintain when you eat intuitively (which few people do because of our diet culture). The set point theory of weight suggests that based on genetic factors, your body wants to be a certain weight, which is the weight that will best keep you healthy based on your specific needs. Some people have a higher setpoint, while others have a much lower set point. It is also important to understand that people will have shifting set points throughout their lives. These changes won't be significant, but older people often gain weight because of metabolic changes that naturally occur. Your body tries to regulate your weight when it is left to its natural devices; thus, while having more weight isn't bad, many people may rise above their set point weight when they are binging, leading to them feeling uncomfortable in their skin and not feeling as energized as they should.

The set point theory comes down to your brain and your hormones, which function together to maintain balance in your body. Your hypothalamus is the part of your brain that is signaled by your fat cells. Your fat cells help your body determine your nutritional needs throughout the day. Hormones, like leptin that helps you feel satiated, and ghrelin, which makes you hungry, will be used by the body based on stimuli it receives and patterns from your daily activities. Naturally, your body lets you know when you need food and when you don't, but when you use a diet, your body's signals are thrown out of whack, which can result in weight gain. Set point theory suggests that when you restrict your food intake, your body will start to focus more on food and slow down your metabolism to maintain its weight.

While not all scientists believe in set point theory, it speaks to the idea that when you were born, your body knew when you were hungry. As a baby, you cried when you wanted food, instinctually knowing that you were hungry. Thus, there's a way to find peace with food now too. You just have to get the cacophony of diet culture out of your head to do so, which, given how many diet ads and unhealthily thin models you see daily, is hard.

Our eating habits are often a game for companies. While over forty-percent of adults are obese and the dieting industry continues to get larger, obesity rates are not leveling off, which shows that very little change is being produced by our diet culture. Rather, companies are exploiting body standards and pressures to make more money. They convince you that you're not happy with the way you are because of your weight. But when dieting doesn't help make you happier, they blame the failure on you being lazy and lacking willpower. The reality is, they are evoking the *exact* reaction that they want.

We live in a culture that glorifies many things that lead to dieting and shame around weight, but we never benefit from these glorifications. After all, they are used against us in advertising because those who cannot embody the glorification are then shamed into giving into unhealthy demands. Don't let these glorifications hurt you any more than they already have. Rise above them.

One of the most poignant glorifications is the glorification of thinness or having muscled bodies. Women tend to be convinced that they need to be thin while men usually are convinced that they need to be more muscular. Both are ideals that countless people can't feasibly reach. Over fifty percent of Americans feel dissatisfied with their current weight. Among women who are of a healthy weight, seventy percent want to be thinner. A stunning eight percent of ten-year-olds are afraid that they will be fat. By thirteen, over half of girls don't like their bodies, and by seventeen, that number goes up to seventy-eight percent.

Our culture glorifies overconsumption. In more than just food, academics such as Kima Cargill suggest that our culture of constantly wanting more leads to imaginative hedonism, which is the idea that we envision the triumphs that certain products can give us but are disappointed when those objects don't give us the happiness we expected. This same overconsumption is rooted in diet culture in interesting ways. While the food industry tries to sell us happiness with addictive foods, the diet industry works symbiotically selling us over consumptive methods to lose the weight binging has put on (or that we naturally have based on our set points).

Moreover, our culture glorifies dieting. Because of the latter two glorifications, the celebration of dieting means that we are unable to live up to the expectations of eating plentifully and being thin. You can't both overconsume and be stick thin, so people are forced to teeter between binging and dieting. With so much body satisfaction, diets start young. One-third of children aged ten to fourteen are on diets. Further, a third of teen boys and more than half of teen girls use dangerous methods to manage their weight, such as restricting their food intake, smoking, throwing up, and using weight loss drugs. Among nine to eleven-year-olds, a reported eighty-two percent of families identified as sometimes or very often engaged in active dieting. These numbers are startling and show the unhealthy Western fixation on dieting itself. Even people who don't need to be dieting are being convinced that it's a normal part of growing up. Not only do we binge on food, but we, as a society, binge on erroneous lies that have been spread about the correlation between weight and eating.

Ironically, our culture glorifies eating as much as it glorifies weight loss. As has been discussed, companies use food against us to make us eat more and to encourage overeating. The issue is not just that they are getting us to eat more, but they are encouraging us to consume foods that are addictive and unhealthy. We are inundated by commercials selling us hyper-palatable foods that can lead to addiction. The advertising targets children, especially, engraining over consumptive eating for the youngest of society. Ads highlighting bulk products for discounted prices and addictive foods contribute to the childhood obesity epidemic that is causing the weights of children to skyrocket and setting them up for a future of dieting. Research has shown that these ads predominantly highlight unhealthy foods. Children who watched over three hours of TV per day are more likely to be obese by fifty percent, showing the role of advertising in the glorification of overeating. People are taught that the more you eat, the better you will feel. This simply isn't true. Food ads link success with eating hyper-palatable foods, but in reality, the companies are trying to get you addicted so that you buy more.

The foods that are heavily advertised are full of simple carbs with lots of unhealthy processed sugar and trans fats. These foods are associated with health issues, and they give people spikes in energy and then crashes, which leads to people wanting more just to keep their energy levels up. Everyone can easily bring to mind a hyper child who has had too much sugar and then crashes shortly later. This same effect happens in adults too. We feel energized for a few hours, and revert back to being exhausted. Many experts suggest that sugar could have the same levels of addiction as opiates, since the processes that occur in the brain are markedly similar. Many people who binge eat may also have chemical dependencies, showing that bingers may have more addictive personalities. When we eat sugar, feel-good chemicals like dopamine are released, and our opiate receptors are opened. Thus, we become more compulsive with our eating and other behaviors. Sugar can lead to more headaches, and hormonal problems. We can also become chemically addicted to it, meaning that when we deprive ourselves of sugar, we may eventually binge on it to lessen the withdrawal symptoms and cravings.

The dieting industry promises us a cure to the problems posed by food companies. The dieting industry is a mammoth industry that is worth seventy-billion dollars as of 2019, which is an increase in revenue despite the growing resistance to dieting because of the body positive movement. Diet culture makes people insecure, while body positivity allows people to stop dieting altogether. No one needs to be on a diet. The bottom line is that the diet industry isn't trying to help you. It's there to keep you trapped.

Diet culture is created to hurt us by keeping us in a cycle of wanting and failing to lose weight. Diets don't work, so companies keep you going on and off diets, making you think that if you have enough willpower that maybe someday one of those diets will work. When you look at the statistics on dieting, it is startling to see how widely diets don't work. Researchers estimate that up to ninety-five percent of diets fail, and people generally regain lost weight within five years. Further, of the five percent who do lose weight successfully, ninety-eight percent match the clinical qualifications of having eating disorders. With this in mind, dieting doesn't do much good for anyone. Your options are to keep diet cycling, have an eating disorder, or make peace with food. I know which one I'd pick if I were in your shoes.

Food is representative of other problems in our lives, and companies know that. Often, we try to control our food as a way to deal with the hardships we sometimes face. I spent years thinking that my weight was the biggest problem in my life when it wasn't! The weight loss commercials not only suggest that using their product will result in weight loss, but also that your whole life will change as a result of losing weight. The truth is, though, your weight doesn't cause you to binge. You binge because of how you feel about yourself, which goes much deeper than your weight. When you feel insecure about your weight, you begin to question your worth as a person, which leads to your relationship with food, becoming even more detrimental to your well-being. Binging is not just about food; it's about your feelings and views of yourself too. Diet culture promises you happiness, but the only way to acquire happiness is to learn to love yourself as you are.

Restriction of food commonly leads to binging. The statistics don't lie. Young girls who go on diets are twelve times more apt to binge eat compared to those who don't diet. When you restrict food, not only does it throw off the chemical processes in your body, it makes your brain think that you are at risk. Your brain begins to worry that you are facing a famine and your body begins to slow down its metabolism to conserve energy. Afterall, your body is wired for survival, so when you try to lose weight, your body will fight you because it is trying to ensure that you stay alive. While famine for most people in the Western world isn't a predominant concern, your body is still used to times in the history of humanity in which famine was a pressing concern. Thus, diets force you to fight your very instincts.

The very way in which people are classified as either unhealthy or healthy shows the gross misunderstanding of how people's bodies work. It's important to realize, therefore, that there are several flaws in how people are classified in their weight groups, which determine how doctors treat patients. BMI, or the scale commonly used by medical practitioners, is a flawed method of determining health. BMI is not a perfect method of seeing how much body fat people have. Muscle weighs more than fat, so people who are muscular may be categorized as obese. A bodybuilder, for example, may weigh the same as someone who is obese but will have very little fat. Unfortunately, BMI continues to be used because doctors are still obsessed with the use of weight as a marker of health, which leads to the discrimination of heavier people in medical practices. To make matters worse, better methods have not been discovered for measuring fat, so while BMI often brings unnecessary shame onto people, it continues to be common in the medical community.

Myths being spread about larger bodies being bad are harmful to eating behaviors and how people function. When a whole society worships thin, even unhealthily thin bodies, it becomes easy to fantasize about whittling yourself down to a smaller size. People constantly stigmatize fat people, who are then made to feel like there's something wrong with them when the real sickness lies with society.

More than anything else, a culture of shaming people for their bodies can have adverse effects on the health and lifestyles of people. The societal pressures could be more harmful than extra weight. While higher BMIs have some association with reduced health, the actual health risks perpetrated may not be caused by the factors people commonly associate with obesity. Various researchers have argued that weight stigma, or the negative views and biases associated with weight, cause many of the health problems associated with being overweight. Common ideas that weight stigma perpetrates are that larger-bodied people are either lazy or simply don't have will power. This bias can be seen in individuals as young as three years old, showing how pervasive this phenomenon is our culture. In a well-known study from the 1950s, children were shown several images of other children and asked to rank them in order of which ones they liked best. The pictures included both "healthy" weight children and obese children. It also showed children with physical disabilities or facial disfigurements. In six groups of children who were of varying classes and races, the obese child came last in the ranking. In the time since that study, weight stigma has only become more deeply rooted in society.

Researchers suggest that it is this stigma that perpetuates the obesity "epidemic." Not only does this stigma make people spiral more out of control with their weight, but it makes them unable to be treated properly.

Additionally, weight stigma causes actual physiological changes in people. In studies, patients who were exposed to weight stigma ate more, were less able to self-regulate their eating, and had increases in cortisol levels (a hormone that is considered an obesogenic). People who experienced weight stigma were also less likely to engage in exercise, making weight maintenance even harder for them. They also have increased chances of mental health issues such as anxiety, being two times more likely to suffer anxiety and mood disorders.

The overall culture of dieting leads to binging, and it also creates great shame for those who binge. It took me years to choose recovery because I didn't realize how normal and societally induced my behaviors were. If there had been greater awareness around the topic and less stigma, I would have been able to share my problems with loved ones sooner and would have had support in getting better before my disorder got worse. You must share your struggles with at least one person in your life. Start breaking the stigma. By defying diet culture, you *can* have a happy and healthy life. It's important to understand, however, that you won't achieve it by counting calories.

Was I Born This Way?

Food and Your Childhood

You may wonder if you were born with your habits or if they were formed by how you grew up. Well, the answer is probably a little bit of both. Your DNA does factor into your binge eating, but your foundational experiences have a role of their own. Some people are predisposed to binge eating disorder based on genetics, but childhood trauma and strife can also be contributing factors. Studies have shown that negative childhood experiences have a considerable influence on eating patterns and obesity. Low-income childhoods as well, for example, can have a huge influence because those who have not had food security may be more likely to binge eat. Therefore, your childhood inevitably shapes your eating habits, so you must learn how your past influences your present. I hope you're ready for a deep dive into when you were a kid!

Examine how your parents treated food because many children learn their eating habits from their parents and carry on those habits into adulthood. Think about how your parents' food habits have been passed onto you or how you have resisted those habits they displayed. It should come as no surprise to you that you might be repeating those same patterns. Perhaps upon recollection, you realize that your dad was a binge eater, or you saw your mom overeating when she was anxious, so you started to eat when you were anxious, as well. These experiences cannot change the eating habits you've established, but they can highlight the areas that are most deeply rooted in your psyche.

Think about a moment when you felt free around food. Maybe you can't remember an *exact* time when you truly felt free with food, but many people can benefit from thinking back to a time when they ate what they wanted without feeling any shame or stigma. Remember how light and joyful you felt back then. Keep that feeling alive as you go through this journey because that's the feeling that you're looking to find yet again. Being mindful of your emotions is the key to progress.

Let go of the negative thoughts that you have internalized. Perhaps, from an early age, your grandma used to tell you that you needed to lose weight. Maybe you were bullied for your weight in school. Maybe you felt like you took up too much space because you were constantly degraded by someone you loved. Whatever negative thoughts that you're carrying, switch them out with positive ones because belittling yourself isn't going to help you stop binging.

Evaluate your eating history. Remember the times it made you feel good, and the times it made you feel bad. Think about when things went wrong with your eating. When did it change? Why did it change? Ask yourself about the emotional attachments that you have to food. In this process, you need to learn your triggers. Do you eat when you're bored? Angry? Anxious? Everyone has experiences that make them more prone to overeating, and many of these have roots in childhood. For example, your beloved aunt may have fed you cookies when you were feeling down, so now, in your adulthood, cookies still pacify you when you feel sad.

Let yourself move on from the past. Don't get stuck in the guilt and shame of things you couldn't control when you were a kid. Children often blame themselves for bad things that happen in their lives, and this blame can lead to continued self-blame if unaddressed. Be merciful with your childhood self. Back then, you were powerless, and you're not to blame for the bad done unto you by other people.

Work through your traumatic experiences. Stop ignoring your past if you haven't yet faced the things that hurt you when you were a child. If you have major traumatic experiences, consider therapy or, at least, find a friend who you feel safe talking to about hardships you've endured. If you still have old wounds, it's terribly hard to move forward, so make peace with what was so you can define what will be.

Know that you are more than your childhood experiences. You're much more than the person you used to be. You've learned, and you've grown. Focus on who you are now and the person you want to be in the future. Never forget the child who you were, but don't get stuck feeling small and helpless. You have the power now, and you can use that power to accomplish whatever you want to accomplish, including putting an end to binging for good.

Your Food Habits

Habits dictate much of what you do on any given day, but for the most part, they are unconscious, so it's easy to go about your day, not even being aware of the things you are doing simply because you're so used to doing them. Habits can be great to have because they allow you to accomplish tasks without having to exert as much mental energy, but when you have bad habits, it's hard to accomplish your goals, and it is easy to default to self-sabotage mode. Therefore, you need to curate food habits that help you move forward rather than walking in place.

Become aware of the habits that you have. The first step to any change is becoming aware of the processes that are normally unconscious to you. Make a list of habits that bother you. It helps to know all the things that trouble you the most. By writing a list of all your habits, you are becoming self-aware, which allows you to take the first step forward in shifting your life. Also, acknowledge the habits that you like. It's always good to look at what you're doing well because that helps keep you in a positive headspace.

Don't let your habits define you. Just because you eat a lot of sugar, doesn't in any way make you a bad person. Your food habits have nothing to do with your character. Moreso, they are related to your DNA and your tastes. Wanting to change something doesn't mean that thing is bad as it is. Wanting to wear a different outfit doesn't mean you hated the last one you had on, and the same can be said concerning healthy eating habits. Instilling more nutrient-dense food in your diet doesn't mean that your old diet habits were bad; it just means that you're making a change that reflects the dynamic needs of your body and mind.

Understand that habits can be changed. Don't let yourself feel defeated just because you have some bad habits. I'll talk more about how to instill good habits later, but the short of it is that habits can be changed. It takes time to change them, which causes many people to give up on changing prior habits when they've only just started making progress. Nevertheless, an old dog can always be taught new tricks, do dedicate yourself to making change because that's the best way to ensure that change will *actually happen*. It also helps that I'm not asking you to make drastic changes. Every habit you swap out will feel relatively easy. Just like you aren't defined solely by your childhood experiences, you don't have to be defined by your habits either, so accept your old habits while embracing your new ones too.

Food and Your Emotions

The hardest part to deal with when it comes to binge eating is your emotional connection to food. You're never going to stop having one, and that's okay, because you don't have to steer clear of the foods that make you feel good. You'll always have memories related to food, and trying to change those memories would be a waste of time.

Even now, after being free from food worries for so many years, I still have an emotional connection to food. I don't let that connection drive my life, but some things cannot and should not be severed. For instance, I still have fond memories associated with my mom's gingerbread dough that we'd roll out and cut into shapes to make dozens of fun cookies. Similarly, chocolate cake with mint icing will always remind me of my dad. I can't help but grin a little when I eat it, although, I would never binge either of those foods anymore. I no longer feel the need to because I've learned to respect the emotional connection I have to food, which allows me to eat in moderation.

It may take you a while to get to where I am. It took me months to get rid of binge eating together, but there are ways you can become more cognizant of your emotional connection to food. Make a list of foods that give you comfort, and these foods should be the first that you stop restricting. Eat them even if it feels scary to do so. Give your body what it wants so that it can get better.

Know that it's okay to use food as a source of joy. Eat things that you love! Make your favorite recipes and share your food traditions with your kids. Having peace with food means that you can love it again. It doesn't have to be something you both love and hate all at once. You can even find new ways to love food. Try foods you've never let yourself taste before. Experiment with new cuisines and take the limits off yourself. You don't need to be uncomfortable around food any longer.

Social experiences shouldn't make you feel nervous just because food is there. Social encounters can be hard when you binge eat because just being around food can make you feel like you're going to lose control. You don't realize how many social events are centered around food until food starts to become the enemy. When I was in college, there were countless times when I blew off my friends just because they were going somewhere that had a lot of food. I couldn't go to a buffet without feeling like I was going to completely lose control over the situation. I stopped enjoying my experiences with the people I loved, and when I did go out with them, my time was ruined by all the worrying I did over food. I felt so disconnected from everyone because I was trapped in my head. It was remarkable how much more engaged I became when I stopped binge eating. It was as if a switch had flipped, and I was finally free to be me again. I could enjoy being social without that constant worry that binge eating might be linked to it. I want you to find the same liberation and be able to go out and have fun.

Trust in your body to make sure you don't go too overboard when you indulge rather than trying to control your eating with restriction. I will warn you that it will take your body some time to realize that you are not going to deprive it. You may have the urge to binge for months after you've started making changes, but that's okay. This is a process, so it's not going to shift overnight. Don't get discouraged if you even gain weight when you first start eating more mindfully because your weight will fluctuate a bit before reaching into its set point.

Food and your emotions will never be fully disconnected, so relinquish the control you're trying to have over your hunger and let yourself experience food without limiting how much you can enjoy it. Nothing should be off-limits anymore because limits only lead to binges.

Chapter 2: Slow Down and Silence The Urge

Eat Slowly and on Purpose

Mealtimes shouldn't be something that you rush through just to get them done. Take your time with meals so that your body can digest food properly as you learn to feel satiated and eat your meals with purpose. Always know why you are eating and give your full attention to the mealtime so that you can upkeep positive habits and look upon meals with positivity and joy. You need to learn to love food again and enjoy every bite you take. If you're not, there's a good chance you are not eating with respect to your body.

Why Eating Slowly Helps

Diet books have long advocated for eating slowly, and there's science backing up how beneficial it can be. While this book has an incredibly different goal than weight loss books, I agree that there are several benefits to eating at a moderate pace. In short, eating slowly can make you feel full faster, and it also helps you break from the typical binge behavior of eating too quickly, which allows you to be more mindful when you are eating.

Eating slowly gives your hunger signals time to kick in. It takes around twenty minutes before your body can recognize that it is full, so by eating slowly, you can better read your hunger signals and be in tune with how much food you need. When you eat too quickly, your body just isn't ready to keep up with you because the necessary processes and release of chemicals takes time.

You digest your food more easily when you eat slowly. Your GI tract works using a step by step process. At the beginning of this process, you begin to salivate when you smell the food or even just think about it. From there, you begin to eat the food, and it starts to break down in your mouth using saliva as well as chewing. As you start eating, your stomach needs to prepare for the food that is coming and prepare digestive acids. Accordingly, if you eat too quickly, you're forcing your digestive system to operate before it is adequately prepared, which is why eating slowly can give your system a better chance at properly digesting your food.

People who eat more slowly feel more content post meals. In a study by the University of Rhode Island, researchers found that women who ate meals faster not only ate more calories, but they felt less lasting satisfaction after eating. So, by eating slowly, you will be able to appreciate your food and feel more satiated until your next meal.

Research suggests that the pace in which you eat matters, so don't shovel all your food into your mouth as quickly as possible when you are eating. Mealtimes don't need to be rushed, so let yourself savor the meal that's in front of you so that you don't wind up binging later when you feel unsatisfied because you didn't get the enjoyment you wanted from your food.

Enjoy Your Meal

If you're not enjoying your food, you're never going to feel satisfied because you are not fulfilling your needs. When I was binging, I never enjoyed my food. I loved the taste of it, but in a binge, I barely tasted anything. The food glided over my taste buds, slithering down my throat before I could even appreciate it. When you're eating at lightning speed and simply trying to get as much food into yourself as possible, you're not focusing on the tastes and textures of what you're eating. You're wasting the experience of eating by not truly enjoying it.

Don't eat foods that you hate no matter how nutritious they are. If you don't like certain vegetables or fruits, don't eat them! Eating foods that you don't like will only make you crave foods that you do like more and lead to binging. Find alternatives for the foods that you don't like so that it never feels like you're forcing yourself to eat anything that you absolutely despise.

Allow yourself treats. When you crave something, eat it. Don't eat it and then punish yourself later by restricting what you have at your next meal. Just eat and don't make a big deal out of the calories or nutritional facts. There's nothing wrong with having the foods that most delight you when the urge strikes. When you let yourself eat these foods, you won't want to binge them because you won't feel deprived. Enjoyment is key in healing from binge eating, so cutting out your favorite treats is counterproductive.

Try new recipes, and don't let your meals become too stagnant. When you eat the same thing every day, meals can get incredibly boring. Thus, you need to try different foods whenever you can. You need to make sure that mealtimes are something you enjoy having. I'm sure that you have enough stress during your day, so you need time when you can relax and enjoy your food. Make it a priority to sit down for meals and savor the food you are eating because it will make a dramatic difference in your progress.

How to Eat With Purpose

Eating should never be something that you do just because. Eat with intention. For each meal you have, you should remain in the moment and mindful of the meal that is in front of you. When you binge eat, it's easy to lose purpose when it comes to meals. You become so used to eating massive quantities that eating stops being special and even feels like a chore at times. Find your purpose in meals to reinvigorate your joy of eating.

Don't eat while distracted. Eating shouldn't be done in front of your TV, and you shouldn't be trying to eat while you work. Eating should be an activity all of its own. It's okay to eat with other people and talk during your meal because that's part of the mealtime experience, but doing activities that distract you from the purpose of your meal isn't helpful.

Make time for meals. We all have busy lives, but you need to prioritize meals. They're incredibly important because meals keep you alive. Don't let yourself skip meals just because you get busy. That's not a good enough excuse. Eat meals and have snacks when you feel hungry between meals. If you want to get better, you have to dedicate the appropriate time to your meals because making sure your hunger is respected as one of the best things you can do for yourself. Respect your hunger by letting it be fed promptly.

Don't be afraid to make meals a social experience. Get your loved ones involved in making mealtimes feel more focused. Eating alone can be triggering and feel like it's not worth the time, so whenever you can, try to bring people you enjoy being around into the experience of eating. Sharing meals is one of the most rewarding activities that humans can do. Breaking bread with others has deep cultural significance, so a meal often feels more like a meal when other people are around. Having other people around helps structure a meal, giving it a beginning and an end, but also, the company of other people can be a great distraction from any troubling food thoughts.

Never count calories. Ever. If you have an app on your phone, delete it right now. There's no reason to keep track of what you are eating that specifically. Not only are people inaccurate when they calorie count, but calorie counting apps will never know the needs of your body, as well as your body does. Don't stress yourself out with numbers that don't even matter. Let yourself be calm and free from worrying about how much you are eating.

Be grateful for what your meal has provided for you. Whatever in life guides you, be thankful for your nourishment and the meal you have. Gratitude is a great tool and allows people to feel more optimistic and have a positive outlook on life.

Remind yourself of all the good things that the food is doing for your body. Food allows you to talk to your friends, work, read, laugh, and a million other activities. Everything you do requires energy, so eat with that purpose in mind. Envision all the things that food will allow you to do. Eating with purpose takes time to master, but it's well worth the effort.

The Benefits of Keeping a Food Journal

Too many people dismiss the usefulness of a journal, but journaling is one of the most helpful daily activities that you can do for a myriad of reasons. Those who journal are better able to make changes in their lives. Not only do people who journal feel better about their situation, they also are overall healthier people. Maybe you doubt how effective journaling is, but let me highlight some of the key benefits, and I'll see if I can change your mind.

Keep in mind that your food journal should be much more than just what you're eating. I also want you to note how you are feeling. Feel free to include things that seem unrelated to food— like an issue you have at work— because even the smallest things can influence your food behavior and lead up to a binge. With that in mind, write as much as your day in your journal as you'd like. The more information, the better.

Journaling has been shown to have several health benefits, and I'm not just talking about mental health benefits. Not only is it a great stress reliever, but journaling for just fifteen minutes three days a week has been shown to lower people's blood pressure. Journaling is also beneficial to your memory. It helps you comprehend the world around you better and also improve your cognitive processing. If that's not enough, those who journal, get sick less often because studies have shown that people who can express themselves through words can improve their immune system. The simple act of journaling can improve conditions such as asthma or arthritis, showing how miraculous utilizing your brain in the right ways can be.

People who journal are also happier. Those who are in the habit of journaling benefit from being able to handle their moods better. People who can be self-reflective can better engage in the world and be more creative in their everyday lives. Thus, journaling leads to people feeling more confident in their skills and creative abilities.

When you keep a journal, you're holding yourself accountable. You're not allowing yourself to put off recovery until tomorrow. You're forcing yourself to live up to what you accomplish. You need that accountability to ensure that you stay in line and don't start fooling yourself. I used to fool myself a lot. I'd convince myself that I could start getting better tomorrow, but then tomorrow came, and I would binge again and vow that tomorrow would be different. It never was until I finally decided that I needed to take charge of my life and stop letting myself get away with hurting myself. I had a moment of realizing that I had to start holding myself responsible for my actions, or I'd be living in binging and dieting torment forever.

Research shows that people who write stuff down are more likely to accomplish goals and complete what they have written down, showing how journaling can influence your mindset. A survey taken by Harvard Business Study shows that eighty-three percent of people have no goals while fourteen percent of people had goals that they didn't write down. Only a mere three percent of people wrote down their goals. Correspondingly, in a study by the Dominican University of California, that groups who wrote down their goals had increased odds of achieving them.

Writing down things such as your food intake and how you feel when you eat can help you identify patterns in your behavior. When you write stuff down, you become conscious of it. Many of our food behaviors are unconscious. We do them out of habit, meaning that we easily lose sight of what we're doing to ourselves. The longer you keep your journal, the more you will learn about yourself. I've had countless moments of realization when writing in my journal. It's almost as good as therapy!

By keeping a journal, you can feel in control of your life without having to manipulate your eating. A journal can be a place to vent all the things that make you feel out of control. You can take the power back by working through your problems instead of continuing to avoid them. Avoidance isn't a tactic you can afford to use anymore. It's time to face up to your feelings and behaviors.

Don't be obsessive about counting calories. The goal of journaling is not to fixate on quantity. I want you to keep your food talk in your journal vague. It's good to write down what you're eating, but instead of quantifying what you are eating, I want you to try qualifying it. Instead of writing, for example, "25 chips- 150 calories," I want you to describe those chips, "delicious kettle-cooked barbeque chips that satisfied my craving." Be honest with what foods you are eating, but be sure to include how you are feeling as well. If you feel unsatisfied with a certain food you've eaten, don't be afraid to admit that. When you binge, write that down. There's no point in lying to your journal or yourself. You're the only one in the world who is going to read it, so don't be ashamed about being honest.

Journaling can be beneficial for anyone, but it is especially beneficial for people who desperately need to promote change in their lives. It takes less than half an hour a day to make meaningful changes in your life through your journal. Even if you're still skeptical, it's worth a shot. It can't hurt, can it?

Instant Gratification Is the Enemy

What Is Instant Gratification?

Instant gratification is receiving an immediate reward for your actions. Many people expect instant results. They want their reward right away rather than waiting for it to come in the future. Instant gratification is one of the reasons why binging feels so good. When you binge, the second that food hits your mouth, you get the great sensation of tasting food that was once off-limits. You don't wait to be gratified, and as you eat, you keep wanting more of that gratification. However, nothing feels as good as that first bite. You become addicted to that first wonderful sensation and keep chasing it as you binge and binge.

The neuroscience behind instant gratification makes sense. Instant gratification gives our brains a different feeling than a delayed reward does, and the delayed reward often doesn't give us the same rush of overwhelming happiness that instant results do. The brain understands immediacy well. If you fall on your arm and your arm is broken, you know why your arm is broken. The pain you are experiencing makes perfect sense, but if you didn't feel that pain until a month later, you'd be a lot more confused about why your arm is hurting. Therefore, it makes sense for us to experience things right away, and it's harder to think in the long-term.

One quintessential experiment nicely shows the role of instant gratification in decision-making. The Stanford Marshmallow Experiment is one of the most well-known experiments of all time. In this experiment, young children around five-years of age were sat in rooms with marshmallows on the table in front of them. The children were told that they could eat their marshmallows right away, but if the children waited until the researcher left and came back into the room that they could have second marshmallows. After leaving the room for fifteen minutes, the researcher came back, and some kids ate the marshmallows as soon as the researcher left the room while others waited a little longer. A few were able to wait the full time. The experiment then followed the children for forty years to find patterns among those who were able to delay gratification and those who weren't.

The children who were able to delay their gratification grew up to have better test scores, were less likely to abuse substances, had better social skills, were less obese, and could better manage stress. Interestingly, these children had been divided into groups, and one group was promised crayons and then never got them while the second group was given the crayons that they were told they would get. The children who had learned that they couldn't trust that they would get what they were promised, tended to eat the marshmallows more often.

The same concepts come into play in binge eating. When you restrict your food intake, your body believes that it is not going to receive the food that it expects, so you binge, and your body is resistant to receiving any delayed reaction. Many people who experience binge eating disorder may have a harder time with impulse control, meaning that instant gratification can seem even more appealing. Research has suggested that overeating is often caused by a lack of long-term thinking, which makes it hard for people to resist the marvelous tastes of food that they could have right now.

Why Is Instant Gratification Bad?

The need for instant gratification can be counterproductive to your progress because it allows your potentially destructive impulses to take control of your actions rather than letting you make clear, controlled decisions. You stop being in control and the instant gratification becomes the decision-maker. Don't let instant gratification be the thing that defines how you behave. You don't need to give in to your impulses. Instead, with a little practice, you can let yourself be future thinking.

Unfortunately, instant gratification causes you to act before you think. You find yourself diving headfirst into a bag of chips before you can think any better of it. I've been there hundreds of times. When I binged, it would feel as though I was in a trance, and I no longer felt like I was making my own decisions. I'd start eating, promising that I'd have just one taste, but then, knowing that I was just going to restrict my food intake again, I kept eating. I figured that

I was already ruining my diet, so I might as well make the most of it. I gave into my immediate urges and rationalized them instead of considering what doing so might do to future me.

Instant gratification also prolongs how long you have to wait to get results. Instant gratification makes you put off lasting change by tearing your focus from your goals. You constantly focus on what you can do to feel good now rather than what you can do to feel good permanently. Instant gratification makes you put things off until tomorrow because you're too focused on what you can receive today.

Instant gratification doesn't give you long-term satisfaction. Binging doesn't feel good. It makes your body ache, your throat hurt, and your lips dry from all the salt and sugar you've eaten. It makes you feel a bit hungover— a headache and nausea overcomes you as the food finally settles. Mentally, you don't feel any better. You feel ashamed and angry at yourself for messing up yet again. You get caught up in a self-pitying spiral, and no matter what you do, you feel disgusted at your behaviors. Binging often feels good as you're doing it, but then the appeal wears off, and you feel worse than you did before.

You'll never accomplish anything in the future if you're only looking at what you can get out of today. You need to stop seeking instant gratification because it will never give you the long-term satisfaction that I'm sure you want. It will be hard, but you can use a few simple tips to help yourself look ahead instead of getting caught up in the moment.

How to Avoid Striving for Instant Gratification

Don't expect results right away. You're not going to stop binging overnight. Your body needs time to adjust to the changes you are making and realize that you are not continuing your unhealthy relationship with food. Once your body feels secure and knows that you are going to take care of it, it will start to fall into place, and you'll have the urge to binge at lessening frequency. In time, you will be free of binging altogether, and your set point weight will be restored.

Visualize the future. Visualization is a great tool to make what you want to happen in the future come true. Psychologists have found that visualization is an impactful technique that anyone can do from the comfort of their own home. High performing athletes, celebrities and billionaires have all used visualization to make their dreams come true. Imagine yourself in the future, holding your favorite food. Now imagine a monster looming behind you, pestering you to eat that food. Visualize yourself, checking in with your hunger, and realizing that you aren't hungry. Finally, visualize yourself telling the binge monster that you don't want your favorite food and hand over the food to him. By imagining what can happen in the future, you're setting yourself up for success and giving yourself a taste of what you can look forward to.

Remind yourself what you're fighting for. Never forget why you want to quit binging. Remember all the agony and discomfort that your binge eating has put you through. Think of your lowest moments and keep remembering not just how far you have to go but how far you have come in your binge eating journey. By remembering what you don't want to go back to, you will have the motivation to carry on, even if the results aren't instantaneous.

Make daily goals. Incremental goals will help you find gratification each day. As you wake up every day, make a to-do list of the things that you would like to accomplish. Keep it simple so that you don't overwhelm yourself, but make sure that you have tasks to check off your to-do list. Completing these small tasks will make your long-term goals feel more manageable. One thing you can do is say, 'I will not binge today," and that seems a lot more manageable than saying, "I will never binge again," right at the start of your journey. Most people can't just stop on day one. If they could, they would have done it by now, so don't expect to *never* binge again. Slip-ups happen, and it's okay.

Find victory in little things. Any progress you make shouldn't be scoffed at or minimized. Not binging for one day when you usually binge every day is an amazing step forward. It may not seem like much, but that's more than what many people do. Know that waiting for the reward will get you the best results and embrace the waiting. Let the journey give you joy rather than just the destination.

Listen to Your Body

The human body is an incredible thing, and your body will give you vital information that keeps your hunger at a manageable level and allows you to eat food without fear, but you have to learn to accept and translate that information based on what your body is saying. You need to be able to evaluate both your health and your hunger if you want to ensure that you are staying on the right track.

Evaluating Your Health

Be aware of the changes happening in your body. Note what makes you feel better and what makes you feel worse so that you can more easily make changes that you can stick to. Keeping healthy is a dynamic experience, meaning that you have to check in with yourself. When your body starts to feel a little bit out of synch, adjust and see what tweaks you can make to make it feel better. Some days your body may be more exhausted than others, for example, and when you are tired, you may be more prone to overeating. Thus, listening to the cues that your body gives you, like yawning and aching, can help you counteract your hunger.

Know your body's limits. Maybe you have a physical ailment or intolerances of certain foods. Keep these ideas in mind so that you don't do anything that makes it harder to stick to good habits. Take care of yourself when you don't feel well. If you have not been running, don't get up and try to run a marathon. Exercise can be a great tool for channeling excess energy, but if you're taking on too much at once, you're only going to get yourself hurt. Be gentle with yourself.

Make sure your nutrition matches your health needs. Certain foods can benefit people with select conditions. If you have any chronic conditions, do some research on foods that can help alleviate some of your pain or other symptoms. Don't restrict anything that your body needs to function. If you're having cravings, they may be a sign of what your body needs. Your body often craves foods that contain essential nutrients, so listen to your cravings when they arise.

Remember that without your health, you can never have happiness. While the way your body looks doesn't matter, how it functions is vital. Your brain can't accomplish what it wants if your body isn't up for it. Your body should be something you value, and when you value your body, you treat it well. You don't put it through unnecessary hardships or ignore its signals. Learn to respect your body and its abilities regardless of what size that body is. As soon as you can do that, you'll be able to accomplish true inner peace.

Evaluating Your Hunger

If you can evaluate your hunger, you will be able to maintain healthy eating patterns without having to use rigid diets that only make you feel worse about yourself and your condition. Understanding your hunger will give you the tools you need to understand what your body requires to function optimally. Learn to observe your hunger cues and to become fully aware of not only that your body needs food, but what *kind* of food it needs. Of course, doing that can seem overwhelming, and it takes extensive practice, but there are several ways in which you can gauge your hunger and get more in touch with your body.

Strive for intuitive eating, but don't let yourself get overwhelmed by expecting to be able to eat intuitively right away. It takes time to transition. Intuitive eating is a concept with several principles that help people get in touch with their hunger signals. Intuitive eating includes people of all sizes and resists diet culture. Intuitive eating allows you to eat whatever you want as long as you are listening to what your body is saying. It teaches you not to see food as good or bad, but to see the gradient nature of food and that any food is okay to eat so long as you recognize when you are full.

Learn to rank your hunger until you can eat intuitively without thought. The use of a hunger scale can help you determine whether your desire to eat is rooted in actual hunger or is a physical need. Commonly, hunger scales rank hunger from a level of one, which is ravenous for food, to ten, which indicates that you feel so sick you can't eat anything more. Meanwhile, a seven would represent when you feel totally satisfied and a level four is when your hunger first begins. The other numbers fall somewhere between. Make a scale with rankings that fit you. You can define what levels of hunger stand out most to you. You can use your scale before and after meals to check in with yourself on what your body needs. Using a scale will help you identify emotional hunger from physical hunger.

The hunger scale method is straightforward, but it can be hard at first because you may be out of touch with your body. But the more you use it, the more natural it will become until you can intuitively know when you need food and when you should stop eating.

An example of a hunger scale is as follows:

1. You're feeling dizzy, shaky, or weak.
2. You're struggling to pay attention and are moody.
3. You're starting to feel uncomfortable because of your hunger.
4. You're beginning to feel hungry.
5. You're currently content, but you could have more food.
6. You're not hungry or full.
7. You're satisfied but starting to get full.
8. You're starting to feel bloated and overly full.
9. Your clothes are starting to feel constrictive.

10. You're so full that you feel sick.

Respect your hunger. Your hunger is something that you cannot change. It exists within you, and not letting that hunger exist means ignoring all the problems associated with that hunger, as well as, all the joys.

Chapter 3:
Improve Your Nutrition, Improve Your Life

What Are My Daily Nutritional Requirements?

There are certain foods you should make sure that you have daily. The World Health Organization has suggested that twenty nutrients are deemed necessary for health, which includes micronutrients, fat-soluble vitamins, thiamine, niacin, riboflavin, vitamin B6, pantothenic acid, iodine, magnesium, zinc, biotin, vitamin B12, vitamin C, calcium, antioxidants, and folate. These are all important for optimal human function, among others.

The nutrients that you put in your body are vital to your health, and if you are not healthy, you will not be able to stop binging. Therefore, learn what foods you should be eating to get all the nutrients you need and learn the pains and problems that may occur when you don't.

The United States Department of Agriculture suggests that people try to find foods that are a modest portion, are nutritionally dense, and are varied. Furthermore, it emphasizes making small, incremental changes to improve your health. Nevertheless, the USDA, just like me, says that our specific circumstances influence what we eat and that each person will have plates that look unique. There are, however, certain foods that nutritionists would urge you to be sure to include in your diet. The first category you need to learn about are macronutrients, which make up the caloric content of your food and give you energy. Macronutrients include carbs, proteins, and fats. Alcohol is a less nutritionally necessary macronutrient that contains seven calories per gram.

Carbs

Carbs are maybe one of the most controversial macronutrients. You can probably identity some foods that contain carbs such as cookies, cake, and bread, but you may be less clear on what a carb is. Carbohydrates, commonly referred to as just carbs, are created using carbon, hydrogen, and oxygen. Carbs have four calories per gram. On average, people need about 135 grams of carbs per day, but each person will have distinctive needs based on their weight and how much energy they use. For example, a diabetic may want to limit carbs to ensure they remain under a certain number while a pregnant woman may require more carbs than average. Generally, you should aim to have forty-five to sixty-five percent of your caloric content be made up of carbs.

You need to have carbs daily unless you are told to cut back for medical reasons (a keto diet, which is a low carb diet, can be used to help people with epilepsy and other disorders in select cases). Your body uses carbs to provide energy to working muscles, as well as your central nervous system. They also make sure your muscles aren't used to fuel your body and allow your fat to metabolize. Carbs are also the preferred energy source of your brain. In the absence of carbs, the body can convert fat into ketones in a process called ketosis, but the body is built to fuel your brain using carbs, making them essential to your body.

Carbs often have a bad reputation in the world of dieting. They are often treated as unhealthy and fattening when that couldn't be further from the truth. What people do not realize is that not all carbs are created equally. There are two categories of carbs: simple carbs and complex carbs. Simple carbs are the carbs that are often vilified by diets. While you shouldn't eliminate them completely from your diet, you should know that these carbs do not make you feel as satiated because they are digested more quickly. Further, simple carbs will lead to your energy levels crashing quickly. They also tend to have reduced nutrition because fiber-filled portions have been removed. Complex carbs, meanwhile, are polysaccharides meaning that they have at least three sugars in them, whereas simple carbs only have two. Complex carbs make you feel energized longer and satiated. Foods such as whole grains, potatoes, and legumes are examples of complex carbs. It is important to add more complex carbs to your diet for better health outcomes. Research has suggested that eating carbs instead of saturated fats can reduce your risk of heart disease and diabetes.

People who do not have enough carbs in their diet will likely feel changes in their bodies. You may start to feel moodier and have trouble concentrating or remembering. When you don't have enough carbs, your decision-making skills may also suffer, making it harder to maintain good dietary decisions as the day drags on. Thus, try to include complex carbs in your diet so that you can feel happy and healthy.

Proteins

Proteins are the macronutrient that people tend to rank with the most fondness, and for good reason. They have four calories per gram. While all macronutrients are important in a balanced diet, proteins are a jack-of-all-trades and help your body carry out an expanse of functions. The jobs of fats and carbs are more focused, while proteins have roles in several processes. Protein is made of nitrogen, which makes the amino acids that form proteins. Some amino acids can be made within your body, while others must be obtained from food sources. The former group is called non-essential amino acids, while the latter are essential amino acids. There are nine essential amino acids that you need to be healthy. All animal-based proteins will contain all nine of these. Eleven amino acids can be produced by your body if you are getting other nutrients that you need.

Dieters and those who want to gain muscle often love protein because protein can be great in helping you gain muscle, but it also has a myriad of other functions. Protein helps your body break down the food you're eating, repair tissues throughout your body, and make enzymes. It is also one of the main building blocks for things such as your bones, skin, blood, hair, and cartilage.

Focus on lean proteins. Chicken, turkey, 90% lean ground beef, beans, lentils, low fat or skim dairy, salmon, tuna, tuna, and egg whites are all examples of lean proteins, which are proteins that have less than ten grams of fat per serving. Proteins can be found in animal products like dairy, eggs, and meat. They also can be found in plant-based products. Foods like quinoa, amaranth, and buckwheat are nearly complete protein sources. Though, the only complete protein source that is plant-based is soybeans, which are found in products like tofu; however, you can use complementary proteins to make up a full protein that has all the amino acids that you need. Certain proteins can be paired together to add up to a full source. There are three groups of plant-based proteins, and from these groups, you must choose two foods from two distinct categories to get a complete protein. You may choose from grains, legumes, or nuts and seeds. Thus, eating black beans with whole grain rice would provide you a full protein serving. Alternatively, oatmeal and peanut butter would also give you a complete serving.

Eat proteins throughout the day. Whereas your body can store fats and carbs to varying degrees, your body does not store proteins. Thus, it helps to eat several meals and snacks throughout the day, each with protein sources. You shouldn't strive to eat as much protein as possible because your body can only use so much. Generally, men should try to have three servings of protein, totaling to six to seven ounces while women, children, and teenagers can aim to have as little as two servings that contain five to six ounces of protein. The amount you need will depend on your activity level. Burn victims, for example, need additional protein because their bodies have extensive reparations to do.

Being deficient in protein can cause several unhealthy effects on your body. When you lack the proper protein, you may suffer from protein-energy malnutrition (PEM). PEM, in severe cases called kwashiorkor, happens when people do not get enough protein in their diet. These people may be getting the proper caloric value that they need but do not have the protein levels needed for their body to function or even process the food that they are eating. It is commonly seen in countries that are experiencing famine, making it hard for people to get balanced diets. It is also common in alcoholics, who get many calories from alcohol and therefore do not have enough protein. Malnourished people, for example, sometimes experience extra swelling in their bodies— in their feet, stomachs, and ankles— because of the dysfunction caused by a lack of protein. Thus, protein is crucial to your health and ability to be healthy.

Fats

Fats are one of the foods that worry people the most. At nine calories per gram, they are the most calorically dense food, which makes people fear that eating fats will lead to weight gain. Like carbs, fats are frequently misunderstood. The bottom line, though, is that your body needs fat to function. Of course, having too much isn't helpful, but without fat, your body won't be able to keep your organs protected. Fat is responsible for giving your body back up energy that it can burn when the energy provided by carbs has run out. When you exercise, you will start burning fat about twenty minutes into your workout.

Your body needs fats for more than just having energy at the ready for when you're running low on carbs. It's also crucial that you have dietary fat so fat-soluble vitamins like K, D, A and E be absorbed. These vitamins help your hair and skin stay healthy, maintain your vision and support your immune system. They also ensure that your reproductive system works, bones are healthy, and help your blood clot properly. In addition to allowing you to absorb vitamins, fat insulates your body and protects your organs. When your body doesn't have enough fat to fuel you, it will start to break down muscle for energy, including heart muscles, which can lead to issues such as heart failure. Disallowing any fat from your diet is ultimately dangerous to your wellbeing. Aim to ensure fat makes up anywhere from twenty to thirty-five percent of your caloric intake and saturated fat makes up under ten percent of your daily calories.

Some fats are better for you than others. Listed in order from least to most healthy, there are three kinds of fats: trans fats, saturated fats, monounsaturated fats and polyunsaturated fats. It is important to focus on incorporating more healthy fats and less of the others.

Generally, you want to avoid trans fats whenever possible. Trans fats do extensive damage to your health. They increase levels of LDL cholesterol in your blood (which is the bad cholesterol) and decrease how much HDL cholesterol is in your blood (which is the cholesterol that is good for you). Trans fats can also cause inflammation, lead to insulin resistance, cause heart problems, and worsen chronic conditions. One startling statistic from Harvard Health suggests that eating just two percent of calories in trans fat correlates to an increased risk of heart disease. While many countries, including the United States, have banned trans fats, companies can still put trans fat into their foods as long as they are less than 0.5 grams per serving. Fortunately, the number of products with trans fats is decreasing. Some foods like dairy and meat may have limited naturally occurring trans fats, which studies have shown to be less harmful than synthetic trans fats (commonly found in microwavable popcorn, vegetable shortening, fast food, and snack cakes).

Saturated fats aren't as toxic as trans fats, but they should be eaten in moderation. They increase LDL cholesterol, which can cause blockages in your body, so too many can be incredibly harmful. They are found in foods like red meat, full-fat dairy, and many highly processed foods. Don't deprive yourself of these foods but swap out this kind of fat as much as you can for a better health outcome. The better your body feels, the easier it will be not to binge.

Monounsaturated fats and polyunsaturated fats are both excellent for your health. To show how good these fats are, research from the 1960s has shown that despite having a lot of fat in their diets, Greek people who followed the Mediterranean diet had decreased risks of heart disease even though fat was an important part of their eating style. The key was that they ate a plethora of monounsaturated fats such as olive oil, avocados, nuts, safflower oil, and sunflower oil.

Polyunsaturated fats are another type of fat that you need to include in your diet because they are essential fats. These fats not only reduce bad cholesterol, but they can increase good cholesterol. They also reduce the number of triglycerides in your blood. Triglycerides are formed when you eat more calories than you need to use. These lipids being in your blood can lead to heart problems and other health conditions when you have too many. There are two predominant types: omega-three fatty acids and omega-six fatty acids. Omega-threes increase good cholesterol and can help your heart rhythm and reduce your chance for stroke. They could also help with conditions such as arthritis. These fatty acids can be found in cold-water fish like tuna and salmon. They are also found in flaxseeds, canola oil, soybean oil, and certain nuts like walnuts. Omega-six fatty acids are also good for your heart, and they can be found in various vegetable oils like safflower, sunflower, or corn oils.

When your body is deficient in fats, you are unable to have the proper energy stores you need to function and unable to appropriately absorb important fat-soluble vitamins. Therefore, you should try to include healthy fats as often as you can in your diet as opposed to less healthy ones.

Micronutrients

While carbs, proteins, and fats are macronutrients, you should be eating every day; micronutrients include vitamins and minerals that you need to be including in your diet to make sure that you are functioning optimally. Compared to macronutrients, you don't need as high quantities of these in your body, but that doesn't make them any less important. Micronutrients are often found in fruits and vegetables. Naturally colorful foods tend to be packed with nutritional value, and the colors of the foods often correlate to what kind of vitamins they contain, so make sure you're eating a variety of foods.

Some people may need more micronutrients than others. Pregnant women, for instance, need many vitamins to stay healthy. Getting vitamins through food is preferable, but supplements can help those who cannot acquire all their vitamins through their meals.

Fat-Soluble Vitamins

These vitamins, as I've already mentioned, need fat to be absorbed. When consumed, they are stored in your body so that you can use them later. Here is a breakdown of these vitamins and how they affect your body.

Vitamin K is found in leafy greens like spinach and kale, broccoli, milk, cabbage, eggs, soybeans, and pumpkin. It helps your blood clot and helps your bones. Without vitamin K, you may have hemorrhaging, and the calcium in your bones may lessen.

Vitamin E is predominantly found in leafy greens, whole grains, almonds (and other nuts), and vegetable oils. It acts like an antioxidant, is good for your cells, and helps with your immune system. If you're deficient in vitamin E, you may experience anemia, weakened muscles, and hemorrhaging.

Vitamin D helps you absorb calcium so that your bones are healthy. It also improves your immune function. Vitamin D is unique in that you can get it from the sun, but using sun protection (which you should be using) will block the rays needed for vitamin D absorption, and colder climates might not get the necessary sunlight for this vitamin.

54

Luckily, it can be found in other foods like fortified milk and cereals. It's also in some fish like salmon and mackerel. Without vitamin D, you may have soft bones and osteomalacia.

Vitamin A is good for your vision and your organs. Deficiency, however, can lead to vision problems, including blindness or night blindness. This vitamin is found in seafood like shrimp, fortified milk, carrots, mangoes, spinach, beef, eggs, and sweet potatoes.

Water-Saluble Vitamins

These vitamins are not stored by the body, so you need to eat them regularly in your diet. There are eight B vitamins and one C vitamin in this group.

Thiamin (B1) is commonly found in pork, fish, and poultry. It is also found in whole grains, nuts, legumes as well as enriched cereals. Thiamin aids in regulating the body's appetite. It also aids in the process of turning carbohydrates into energy. When you don't have enough of thiamin, you may get a condition called beriberi. As a result, you could have muscle weakness, edema, heart irregularities, and mental fogginess.

Riboflavin (B2) is a vitamin that also helps process carbohydrates as well as fats and proteins. It also ensures that your skin is healthy, and your vision is clear. It is found in dairies like milk, cottage cheese, and yogurt. It is also found in leafy green vegetables, meats, and enriched foods. Without this micronutrient, you may experience eye issues, tongue discoloration, and light hypersensitivity. One tell-tale sign of a riboflavin deficiency is skin problems in the nose and mouth areas.

Niacin (B3) is yet another one that helps with the release of energy. It also helps keep your skin clear, as well as, keeping your nerves and digestive system functioning at their best. Even more importantly, it allows you to create your sex hormones and stress-relieving hormones. You can get this vitamin through most protein sources like meat, fish, eggs, whole grains, enriched cereals, and peanuts. While niacin is not in all these foods directly, your body can convert the amino acid, tryptophan, into niacin. Without it, you may experience a condition called pellagra and have a loss of appetite. You may also experience delirium, flaky skin, be moody, and have indigestion. Most people in the developed world do not experience this deficiency. However, alcoholics may experience it more often.

Pantothenic Acid (B5) can be found in a wide range of foods such as broccoli, mushrooms, chicken, or whole grains, and you need it for fatty acid synthesis to occur. People usually don't become deficient in this nutrient, but in cases when people don't get enough, they might have trouble sleeping, feel sick, and be tired.

Pyridoxine (B6) is generally referred to as B6, and it helps you use carbs that your body has stored. This vitamin not only helps to energize you, but makes more red blood cells that your body needs.

Biotin (B7) helps you metabolize fatty acids. Like many B vitamins, it also helps you process energy. It is found in many foods such as eggs, soybeans, and fish. When you are deficient in this vitamin, you may feel depressed, have muscle pain, and experience a reduced appetite.

Folate (B9) is found in fortified cereals, dark green vegetables, black-eyed peas, chickpeas, citrus fruits, and melons. This vitamin helps keep your red blood cell levels where they need to be. It also aids in protein metabolization and cell division. Without this vitamin, you may have increased odds of heart attack, stroke, or cancer. You may also have heartburn and diarrhea.

Cobalamin (B12) is found in animal products like eggs, meat, and dairy. It is also in fortified cereals. B12 is a critical vitamin as it keeps your brain and nervous system running, while also helping your red blood cells form. Vegans and some vegetarians may need to turn to supplements to ensure that they are getting B12 in their diets. Those who are deficient may feel exhausted and have nerve degeneration, which can culminate in paralysis.

Vitamin C (ascorbic acid) is known mostly for being in foods such as citrus fruits, but it can also be found in dark green vegetables and tropical fruits like mangoes, strawberries, cantaloupes, or papayas. This vitamin helps your body create collagen, which helps heal injuries and maintain bone strength. It also helps you absorb iron while working as an antioxidant that allows you to be more impervious to infections. The deficiency of this vitamin is called scurvy, which is notorious for impacting sailors in the 1700s who did not have proper nutrition while away at sea. Scurvy can cause emotional effects, such as depression and hysteria. It can also cause dental issues, increased odds of infection, impaired wound healing, and muscular problems.

Back to Basics – The Five Food Groups

Micronutrients should be consumed every day. If you make sure to have fruit and vegetables of varied types with your meals, you'll get most of the nutrients you need. Doing so makes it easier not to binge, and you'll feel a lot better.

Vegetables

Vegetables are one of the most important parts of your diet. They contain a high number of nutrients, but they are low-calorie options. You should have around two and a half cups of vegetables a day. Mix up the kinds of vegetables you eat because the more kinds you eat, the more diverse nutrients you will get from what you are eating. Unfortunately, most Americans do not get the required amount of vegetables.

Dark green vegetables and cruciferous vegetables are some of the most nutrient-dense vegetables. In this group, you have vegetables like broccoli, spinach, kale sugar snap peas, cauliflower, lettuce, and cabbage. Red and orange vegetables also are packed with nutrients and include peppers, tomatoes, carrots, and sweet potatoes, while starchy vegetables are more caloric and include potatoes, peas, and corn. Beans and legumes are sometimes categorized as vegetables, but they may also be called proteins. These beans and legumes include black beans, chickpeas, black-eyed peas, and lentils.

Use vegetables in your diet in creative ways. Cook them or eat them raw. Whatever you do, adding some more vegetables won't hurt, and it's hard to eat too many of this food group. Eating vegetables is not only a great way to make you feel full, which will help you not binge, but vegetables have also been shown to reduce people's risks of having heart disease.

Fruits

Fruits are a great, sweet choice to make you feel satisfied with your meal long after it has finished. Apples, for example, have been shown to have great health benefits. Apples, like many fruits, are high in fiber, which can make you feel satiated (more on that soon), and studies have shown that people who ate apples before their meals ate fewer calories. Apples have also been linked to reduced chances of stroke, lower cholesterol, and could even prevent cancer. Apples are just one of the many amazing fruits that can change your life.

According to the USDA, there are two subgroups within the fruit food group: whole fruit and fruit juice. It's preferable to eat whole fruits rather than fruit juice. Fruit juice may not have as many nutrients. Additionally, some fruit juices have a lot of added sugar, so if you opt to have fruit juice, try juices that are 100% fruit juice. You probably know many examples of fruits, but just to be thorough, fruit includes apples, mangos, grapefruits, raisins, and melons.

You should aim to have around two cups of fruit a day (one apple, as a reference, is about one and a half cups). While fruit does have sugar, it is a good natural sugar that doesn't have the same energy spike and crash of the sugars you see in sweets.

Grains

In your diet, you should aim to have about six ounces of grains per day. Grains can taste very satisfying and help satiate you. There are two groups of grains: whole grains and refined grains. Whole grains are grains that have the bran and germ of the grain intact while refined grains removed those two parts, leaving only the endosperm. The germ and the bran contain nutrients like B vitamins, fiber, and minerals; thus, by eliminating parts of the grain kernel, refined grains do not do as much for you nutritionally. The endosperm primarily contains just protein and carbs. Whole grains include whole-wheat bread, popcorn, oatmeal, and brown rice, while refined grains refer to white bread, pretzels, normal pasta, and grits.

Proteins

You already know how important proteins are, so much so that they are their own food group. Eggs and meat are a great source of protein. It can be found in nuts, soy, and seeds as well. Generally, people need around five and a half ounces of protein per day. Nutrition experts recommend that you have a variety of proteins in your diet.

Dairy

Finally, the last food group is dairy. This group includes milk, cheese, and yogurt. It's recommended that you choose low fat or fat-free dairy products whenever possible and that you have three cups of dairy per day. You may use dairy substitutions to get similar benefits (such as nut milk or soy milk).

The Dangers of "Bad" Foods & How They Affect You

Do You Eat "Bad" Foods?

With thousands of articles talking about foods that you should never eat, it can be confusing to figure out what foods are good for you. It's natural to want to classify foods as bad or good because doing so helps you feel less lost when it comes to your nutrition. By labeling foods good and bad, though, you start to employ black and white thinking. Accordingly, you start to categorize foods as things you should eat and things you shouldn't eat with no moderation. This mindset sets you up to binge because it makes you feel deprived. It's time to consider that you may demonize certain foods that don't deserve to be demonized. Now that you know more about nutrition, it should be clear that foods aren't bad or good; they're just different.

Ask yourself if there are foods that you put off limits and examine why you put them off-limits. Do certain foods always lead to a binge? Do you have "binge" foods versus "diet" foods? Are you scared that certain foods would cause weight gain? Identify why you judge foods as bad, and now, let me debunk why those foods aren't bad.

"Bad" Foods Lead to Restriction

The Minnesota Starvation Experiment expertly shows the impacts of restriction on eating behaviors. In November 1944, the University of Minnesota had thirty-six men, who were conscientious objectors to the war, take part in a thirteen-month experiment. These men were first put through a control period in which they were eating a normal amount of food, then a period in which the men were in a state of semi-starvation. The experiment concluded by observing their recovery period in which they increased their calorie intake. Scientists had wanted to also include a phase of starvation, but they could not continue with the experiment because even with a diet that was only restricted down to 1600 calories, the men faced severe psychological ramifications such as becoming suicidal, causing researchers to have to stop the experiment before they could study the full effects of starvation.

The results of this experiment were shocking and became foundational in the understanding of eating disorders. Even with just semi-starvation, the men's psychological states shifted drastically. Some men became despondent, while others became indifferent. Many were moody. They also experienced physical weakness, lowered body temperatures, and slower heart rates. Even their sex drive decreased because of being hungry. Some men were driven to the point of madness. More importantly, men became obsessed with food. They'd think about it even when they weren't at meals and talk about food during much of their free time. They dreamt about food and fantasized about it. They chewed a lot of gum to get the sensation of eating. Some even began to smoke more. They became more detached from social settings, and at mealtimes, they'd become protective over their food. They were starving and setting themselves up for extreme food behaviors when they finally could normally eat again.

As the men returned to normal eating, they became prone to binging. They'd eat what would be several normal meals at one time, causing stomach pain and headaches. During the refeeding process, many binge ate, and some would even purge the food they'd eaten in various ways. They felt ravenous, and they had increased concerns about their bodies. They didn't like to discard any food during refeeding, even if they were full. Many men felt emotionally worse during the refeeding, and they only seemed to feel positive when they talked about food, hunger, or even their weight. Further, some would go to desperate measures to get more food and would even look through the garbage for something to eat because they felt so exorbitantly hungry. Even after months of being able to eat sufficient levels of food, participants carried on their refeeding behaviors, showing the long-lasting impacts of deprivation.

Many diets endorse calorie counts that are equal to low semi-starvation numbers that the men in this experiment had to stuck to, so if you're choosing to utilize those fad diets, you are probably not getting the food you need to feel mentally okay. If any of the behaviors or side-effects experienced by men in the Minnesota Starvation Experiment sound familiar, you are probably in a binge-restriction cycle, and it's not a healthy place to be. You'll never lose weight using that method as much as you may want to, and you will never feel at peace with food.

You need to keep in mind that physiological and psychological restriction each have the same influences on your brain. Whether you physically are restricting or are just mentally restricting, you are *still restricting.* Just the act of thinking that you need to be dieting can cause you to feel deprived, which will result in your brain becoming fixated on the things you tell yourself are "bad." Calling foods bad foods puts you in the mindset of restriction, which will lead to your binge eating behavior when you allow yourself to eat again.

Restriction Leads to Binging

Binge eating is commonly caused by a restriction of some sort. Maybe the restriction wasn't your choice, such as in instances of food insecurity caused by poverty. Unfortunately, the amount of people who have food insecurity is up to fifteen percent, and nearly twenty-five million Americans live in food deserts, meaning food is harder to access because food stores are at least a mile away. Thus, economic factors can also make people feel deprived and be more likely to binge. Psychological deprivation often plays a role as well. In either scenario, when people feel like they are being deprived of food, they start to fixate on food like the men in the starvation experiment. When they finally allow themselves to eat a normal meal, they cannot stop eating because their bodies want to stock up on energy while they can.

Too many people follow a binge restriction cycle. The cycle usually starts with dieting. A person will limit their intake in hopes of getting healthier or losing weight. This restriction will then cause mental turmoil. You will start to crave all the foods that you can't have and be extra ravenous because you feel hungry. Then, to relieve the tension from not eating and alleviate the obsession, you will binge, and it may start as just one meal, but you will decide that since you are already "ruining" your diet that you might as well eat everything you didn't allow yourself to. You end up making your "cheat meal" count to the fullest before you try dieting again. After your binge, you will probably feel guilty for your behavior, which will make you feel insecure and worthless. Those with eating disorders such as bulimia may resort to actions such as the use of a laxative, exercise, or vomiting. The guilty feelings then lead people back into restricting again, making the binge-restrict cycle start anew.

The binge-restrict cycle ultimately doesn't do anyone any good. You always start right back where you started and are filled with guilty feelings. This process is driven by black and white thinking that perpetrates that there are bad foods and good foods. To get better, you need to break those barriers.

Food isn't Bad or Good... It Just Is

While foods have different nutritional levels and it is good for your body to have nutrient-dense food, having the occasional piece of bacon or glass of full-fat milk isn't going to kill you. Food should be joyful, and while I want you to start choosing healthy foods just because they'll make you feel more energized and improve the overall condition of your body, I don't want you to eliminate anything. All the rhetoric about cutting foods from your diet is unhealthy. Some people even suggest cutting great dietary sources like wheat! Of course, it would make sense to avoid foods that you are intolerant too, and many people are intolerant to milk and gluten, but don't eliminate anything just because someone told you it was unhealthy. You need food to live, and it is always okay to eat it if you're hungry and remember that eating bad foods sometimes is much better than not allowing yourself to eat. Your body needs energy primarily to complete the most basic functions. Therefore, consider how much nutrition the foods you're eating have, but don't classify foods into good and bad.

How to Respond to Emotional Eating With Healthy Options

Emotional eating can feel out of your control, but you can take steps to remedy this lack of control by understanding why you emotionally eat and how to choose healthier options. It's not easier to address your emotional eating because you've probably become so used to it that you've forgotten the root causes. However, when you put your emotional eating under the microscope, you should be able to find some enlightening patterns, which you can use to then make changes.

Emotional eating is your tendency to respond to your feelings by eating food instead of addressing your feelings. Thus, you need to know what triggers your emotional eating. Log in your journal times when you feel like eating and what emotions you're feeling during those times. It's good to know what feeling makes you binge because, with this knowledge, you can resist the binge and seek out healthier options when you know you're being tempted by emotional hunger rather than physical hunger. Some of the common causes are boredom, stress, anxiety, and bottled up emotions.

Be able to determine what is emotional hunger and what is physical hunger. Emotional hunger will often be triggered instantaneously by a negative feeling or even a good feeling while physical hunger will happen in gradients. You'll start feeling slight physical hunger before it hits you full force. Emotional hunger will also be linked to comfort foods that you turn to when you're feeling upset. Furthermore, emotional hunger doesn't stop when your stomach is full, while physical hunger does have an end. Know the differences between these two hungers to have better control over your eating.

Learn to enjoy treats. I always used to shame myself for having sweets or junk food. I told myself that I was too fat to have those things. As a result, I'd feel even worse about myself and eat even more than I would have just to fill that emotional hole in my stomach. When you have ice cream or other treats, savor them. Don't gulp them down in one bite. Take your time and appreciate the goodness you are eating.

Have snacks with you whenever you can. That way, if you start to feel hungry, you can tend to your hunger before it gets ravenous. When you're going to work, for example, don't just pack a lunch. Have a couple of snacks handy so that when you get home, you feel well-nourished and don't want to eat everything in your pantry. Avoid that feeling of deprivation altogether so that you can more easily handle recovery from binge eating.

Talk to yourself with kindness rather than with negativity. Using positive self-talk can go a long way in helping to tame your emotional eating. Too many people degrade themselves and have a constant loop of negative self-talk. You don't need to be your own worst enemy. Be kind to yourself and give yourself the encouragement and support that you need to thrive.

Go for a walk. Walking is great for your cardiovascular health, and it can be a meditative experience. Plus, it is not too taxing on your body. You can do something as simple as walking around your neighborhood or even just walk around your house for a while. I prefer nature walks, but wherever you walk, is up to you. Walking is one of my favorite activities when I'm feeling overwhelmed by emotions because it helps me slow my brain and think my actions through. It's worth a try for you too.

Meditation can be an ideal way to help you work through negative emotions and get back in touch with your body. Take some time to close your eyes, focus on your breathing, and become one with your body. You can use guided meditation video or audio, but the process of merely sitting down and breathing counts as meditation. It only takes five minutes a day to put you in a good headspace.

Find a way to relax that you can turn to nourish your feelings. Embrace your feelings rather than running away from them. Hobbies can be great ways to channel your feelings into something constructive. Creative activities like fiction writing or constructing models can let you work through your feelings while making you feel like a success rather than failure.

Dance around your house to your favorite song. This is a simple task, but it can make a stark difference. Play music you like and let your body sway to the music. Music and dancing can send feel-good chemicals through your body and be a good outlet for many people. You don't have to be a great dancer to move or even have rhythm. Just enjoy the sound and the motion, and you are doing it exactly right.

Talk to a loved one. Your friends and family probably want to do whatever they can to make sure that you are happy and healthy. Let them help! Be sure to set boundaries so that they don't add more stress to your life but call a friend when you are feeling emotional or send a text to your mom. Communicating with others is a great way to stop a binge because binges are secretive and isolating.

Find a professional to talk to when all else fails. It's okay to need more help. Many people may need a neutral party to talk about their issues and to help them curb emotional eating. There's nothing wrong with needing a boost from a profession. I saw a therapist when my binge eating was at its worst, and she helped me see patterns and behaviors that would have taken me much longer to notice, and I still seek treatment if I am struggling, though not as often.

By choosing healthier practices over emotional eating, you can learn to stop binging forever. It doesn't take major changes in your life to make the necessary swaps either. It's most important that you are willing to leave dieting behind and ready to choose enriching activities.

Chapter 4:
Create a Winning Strategy to Curb Overeating

Reduce Stress & Anxiety – Choose to Rest & Relax

Reducing stress and anxiety is important because stress and anxiety make you more likely to binge. When stressed or anxious, people are more likely to choose high-fat foods. According to the American Psychological Association, thirty-eight percent of Americans have reported eating too much because of stress. Half of these people said that they were overeating every week or more frequently. Without a doubt, ongoing stress influences the behaviors of many people. Further, your body is more likely to store fat when you are stressed. It's easier to let emotional eating overtake you when you feel that worried feeling in the pit of your stomach. Thus, taking care of your stress is one of the best ways to take care of your binge eating. Here are some ways in which you can choose to rest and relax rather than letting the chaos of your life drive you.

Avoid pushing yourself too hard. Many overachievers tend to want perfection from every area of their lives. I used to beat myself up over getting a ninety-nine on a test simply because I used academic achievement to alleviate the overall anxiety that I felt. We all want to succeed, and there's nothing wrong with ambition, but if you push yourself past what you can feasibly do and expect yourself to never mess up, you're in for a lifetime of worry. The more you try to control things you can't control, the less in control you'll have, so stop trying to dictate everything that happens in your life and learn to live with the uncertainty.

One of the best things that I did to alleviate my stress is I bought a stress ball. It's a little step to make your anxiety better, but it made a huge difference. You can get them for just a few dollars, and whenever you're starting to feel overwhelmed, you can squeeze them and let out some of the tension in your body. I still keep one beside me when I'm working or feeling otherwise anxious. Whenever a surge of anxiety strikes, I can squeeze my worry away.

Having a pet can be another great way to reduce stress. While pets can cause stress of their own for some people (especially if you have a brand new puppy that you have to train), animals are generally therapeutic. Physical touch can help alleviate stress (including human to human touch), so animals can provide a connection to another living creature that feels good. Petting your cat or dog can make you calm down, and having to care for a pet can make you focus on the needs of another being rather than worrying about everything else in life. My cat, Pearl, always makes me feel calmer (even when she's not in an affectionate mood), and just having her around makes me feel less lonely when my husband isn't home.

Disconnect from technology. If you're finding yourself getting too emotionally connected to your phone, put it away for a while. You don't need to be constantly checking in with work while you are at home. It's okay to need time away, and it's okay to put your phone on do not disturb. If you get text messages, it's okay not to answer right away. Sometimes, you need distance from the technology in your life that so distracts you and piles on even more stress. Technology can feel stressfully inescapable, but always remember that you choose when to turn your devices on.

If you do choose to use technology to relax, use it wisely. Social media, for example, is probably not the best idea because it can often cause you to compare yourself to others, which might make you feel even more stressed. Watching a fun comedy or reading a book on your ebook reader may be a great method to relax, but make sure you're not constantly checking your work email as you engage in these activities. The goal is to keep work at work and your personal life personal. By having some degree of separation, you can find spaces in which you can relax so that stress doesn't always loom.

Eat foods rich in potassium. While all nutrients are important, potassium especially can help relieve stress. Foods like bananas or potatoes can help normalize your blood pressure and make you feel more energized. Research has shown that potassium can ameliorate the health risks of stress, such as heart attack or stroke. Thus, while it may seem contrary for a binge eater to use food to relax, staying well-nourished can help your stress levels tremendously.

Listen to music. Any kind of music will help reduce stress, but classical music is known to cause extra significant changes. Whatever music you choose will send dopamine and other feel-good chemicals through your body. Play songs you love, and don't be afraid to sing along. Music can allow you time to escape your worries and have fun. Going to concerts is another suggestion that might help. Live music not only makes you feel good, but it makes you feel like you are part of a moment.

Take a trip. Vacations give you a chance to disconnect from your responsibilities—even just a weekend trip to somewhere close by can make you feel better. When you take a trip, you get to escape from your real life. You get to do things that you want to do rather than things that you feel like you have to do. Go to places that make you feel inner peace. I love weekend trips to my favorite Rhode Island beach, especially when it's first starting to get chilly in the fall. When I stand in front of the beautiful ocean with fog hanging over the water and sand, I can't help but feel I'm in a happier place. Find spaces that make you feel that same way.

Organize your life. Take control of things that you can control rather than worrying about what you can't. Most of what you worry about is out of your control, and that's why you worry about it. It is important to find projects that you have actual control over. You can easily organize your desk or sort through your junk drawer. By taking charge of disorganized spaces, you are defeating chaos, which feels incredibly cathartic. Focus on what you can do because anything else isn't worth your time.

Try crafting. Activities like cross-stitching, crocheting, or knitting can help release some of your anxiety. Plus, crafting will give you a chance to make some cool stuff that you can feel proud of. There's a craft out there for everyone; you just have to find it. When I decided to stop binging, I resumed knitting after years of not doing it, and it felt great to bring that hobby back into my life. Plus, it gave me a way to focus my brain without having to think too hard about all the things that were worrying me.

Start an herb garden or plant other plants that you love. Herbs are good for the air in your house and are purifying, but many also have properties that alleviate stress and anxiety. Researchers have discovered that being close to plants can help you relax. Research from Washington State University shows that stressed people experienced a drop in blood pressure when near plants. Some commonly used herbs to reduce stress are lavender, chamomile, and jasmine. If you don't want to tend to plants, getting a candle, or even just having tea can have a good impact.

Do things for yourself. This suggestion seems a little bit "duh," but doing things for yourself is a powerful statement to your body. Your brain will get the message that it should relax when you treat yourself gently. Take a bath, go to the spa for a day, or take charge of your skincare regime. Whatever it is that you consider self-care, do that. Treat your body with the attention it deserves and reassure it that it doesn't have to worry.

An easy act you can do to relieve stress is chew gum. One Australian study in 2008 showed that chewing gum could lower cortisol in your saliva, which is a stress hormone. Plus, gum can give you the sensation of eating, which is helpful for those of us who like to eat to distract us from our woes.

Make sure you are taking deep breaths. We all need to breathe, and we do it naturally, but our breaths can become shallow when we are stressed, so be sure to make the effort to take especially deep breaths when you are feeling stressed or anxious. Calming breaths can help tame your body's reactions to worry and make you feel better in the process.

Laugh a lot. Laughter has been found to have many health benefits. Not only does it lower stress hormones, but it can also increase good cholesterol levels. Laughing also allows you to fake it until you make it. Maybe you don't feel happy, but by laughing, you will start to feel happy the more you laugh. Watch comedies, talk to a funny friend, browse memes on the internet. Find ways to laugh even if you're feeling awful because the adage that laughter is the best medicine is accurate.

Become Friends With Fiber & Protein

As you know, diet is vital to being able to stop binge eating. The foods you eat can help you curb your overeating, but I want you to focus on fiber and protein. These are some of the foods that will make you feel the most satiated and therefore make you less likely to binge. Fiber and protein should become good friends of yours going forward because they will set you up for success in ways that other foods don't.

Fiber

Fiber is often underestimated by people in how important it is, but those who have a lack of fiber probably aren't feeling as great as they could be. Plus, those who don't have enough fiber may have bowel issues and satiety issues, meaning that adding some more fiber to your diet can change the way you eat and digest food.

Fiber is a type of carb, but it is not one that can be digested by your body, meaning that calories from fiber do not get used for energy. Usually, it's recommended that people have twenty-five to thirty-eight grams of fiber per day, but this number varies based on your size and metabolism. There are two types of fiber that you need to be aware of. They are both important, but they are processed differently by your body and are used for distinct functions. The two types are insoluble fiber and soluble fiber. Soluble fiber can be dissolved by water. It can also be metabolized as it goes through your digestive system. Insoluble fiber does not dissolve in water.

Another perk that fiber has is that it feeds your gut floras, which are good bacteria in your gut that help with various functions that your body couldn't otherwise do. These floras reside in your digestive tract, and they help control your blood sugar, weight, immune system, and they even have a part in brain operations. Trillions of bacteria are in your gut, and they all have unique purposes. Your body isn't able to digest fiber, but the bacteria can digest fiber to use it for better purposes!

Fiber takes up more room in your stomach, which means that whenever you eat fiber, you will feel fuller. Thus, just a little bit of fiber can go along way. Fiber is not the kind of food that you'd want to binge on because it would leave you in pain. When eating fiber, you are more likely to feel satisfied with a modest portion.

Research has shown that having ample fiber in your diet makes you eat less during your meal. Even though fibrous foods are low in calories and full of water, they make people feel more satiated. Apples, as we've discussed, cause people to eat less during meals. This impact has been found in other foods like lettuce as well. In studies of obese women, eating foods that have a lot of fiber resulted in the women feeling less hungry than when they had foods that had a lot of fat.

Be sure to gradually add fiber to your diet. If you increase your fiber levels too quickly, you will have gut pain and bowel issues that will make you uncomfortable. Because of the function of fiber and how bacteria eats it, you may have gassiness if you increase fiber too quickly. If you take your time introducing fiber, this will not be as much of a problem, so try to incrementally add more fiber into your diet until you have the required amount. This is not something that you should try to fix overnight, and your body will have to get used to increased levels of fiber.

Whole foods are often high in fiber. Try to eat many fruits and vegetables, which are low-calorie options that are packed with fiber. Do not remove the skins of fruits whenever possible because the skins often contain the fiber you need. Additionally, you can incorporate whole grains for improved gut function and satiety.

Without fiber, your digestive system simply won't thrive. Those who don't have enough fiber may have stomach discomfort and constipation, which no one wants. The research has long shown that adding more fiber to your diet can make you healthier. Plus, fiber has a myriad of health benefits that allow you to stay full longer without having to eat more food. A companion nutrient of fiber is protein, which has its own abilities that will help you stop binging and only eat as much food as you need.

Protein

We've already talked a lot about protein, but it deserves an extra spotlight because changing my relationship with protein helped me change my life. I'd never been much of a protein eater before. I'm a vegetarian, so I have to think outside the box when it comes to protein and ensure that I am getting all the amino acids I need. Nevertheless, when I started adding more proteins to my diet, I felt tangible changes. I had fewer thoughts of binging, and I didn't feel as though I had to eat so much. While my evidence is anecdotal, scientific studies have shown how helpful protein can be.

One clinical trial by Latner and Wilson from the International Journal of eating Disorders studied the impacts fo protein in women with bulimia nervous or BED, both conditions characterized by binge eating. The women were split into groups and given high-protein or high-carbohydrate foods three times a day over two-week timeframes. Patients who ate the high protein meals were less likely to binge than those who had lots of carbs or the base groups. Those who had the protein only binged, on average, just over one time a week while those in the control group binged around three times a week. Furthermore, those who had protein ate less food at mealtimes and said that not only were they fuller, but they had less hunger as well.

Protein is also good because it takes more energy to digest it compared to other macronutrients. Thus, it takes more for your body to digest protein, which means that increased levels of protein will stay in your system longer while carbs and fats won't be as sustainable. Protein will leave you very satiated, and amino acids found in protein let your body know that you are eating food. It tells the hypothalamus gland, which controls your appetite, that you're not starving.

Another positive aspect of protein is that it encourages fat loss. Instead of losing muscle, having more protein will make it more likely that you lose fat. Those looking to build strength will, therefore, benefit from protein intake without having to use means of restriction to improve their health. While weight loss shouldn't be the goal, protein can help with weight management for those who have had issues with fluctuating weight.

Create a Plan That Helps You Achieve Your Goals

Why You Need to Plan

A plan gives you direction and tells you what to focus on. You have to decide where you want to go with your plan and how you want to get there. Your plan is like a GPS; it tells you where to go on your journey as you steer yourself through the terrain presented to you. You have to fill in what stops you want to make along the way, but your plan will connect the dots for you so that you don't get lost as you get more into your journey.

Planning makes it easier to decide under pressure. When you have a plan, you have the focus you need to make decisions even under stress. You'll be able to choose a healthy snack right now over binging later with a plan. Planning gives you security because it reassures that you can handle your situation no matter how difficult it becomes.

Further, plans save you time. You have less to figure out along the way if you already have a good idea of what you want. You might as well determine what you want before you try to go for it. Otherwise, you'll waste time aimlessly wandering when you could be making strides to ending your binging for good.

How to Create a Good Plan

Decide what goals are most important to you. Also, create mile-markers along the way. If you want to stop binging by Christmas, write that goal down, but also have quantifiable mile-markers along the way. For example, say that you aim to cut down your binging by half midway to Christmas. Your goals can be customized to your interests and how quickly you can reasonably see progress. Be sure, however, that you're not trying to get from point A to point Z without any in-between goals or milestones.

Let your plan have flexibility. Too much rigidness puts you right back into an unhealthy mindset. Journeys often come with detours, but just like a GPS, be able to recalculate your direction and adapt to the terrain you're facing in the present. We cannot predict the future, so things happen, and plans change. Thus, allow your plan to be dynamic. Don't be so set on a specific path that you refuse to find new paths that might work better.

Acknowledge what you are good at and what you are not so good at so that you can react accordingly. Utilize your strong areas in your plan to undermine the areas in which you are not so good. Maybe you're good at resisting binging around other people but binge a lot during the holidays. In this case, you could plan to be around a lot of people during the holidays and make sure that you're never left alone for too long.

Let mealtimes be joyful but focus on nourishment over emotional hunger. Make sure your plan includes all the nutrients you need and make sure that it accounts for the joy that hunger can give you. Don't cancel Thanksgiving dinner because you're afraid that it will ruin your progress. Work it into your plan and learn to live with it.

Be realistic with yourself. Know that sticking to the plan won't always be easy, so don't expect your plan to unfold faster than is logical. Know yourself and use your past experiences to judge what your limits are and how much you can accomplish in a certain amount of time. Don't aim to end binging eating for good tomorrow with no looking back. You'll face a few steps forward, but you will also take a few steps back sometimes. That's part of progress.

Stop the Yo-Yo Diet & Create Healthy Habits

Yo-Yo Dieting, Oh No!

Yo-yo dieting refers to weight-cycling, which is the process of losing and gaining the same weight. It can be seen in many bingers who go between restricting and binging. While it may seem harmless, it can be bad for your health. Not only does it lead to a more weight gain in the long term, it also often causes a higher body fat percentage and loss of muscle. It can also contribute to conditions like type two diabetes and liver issues because yo-yo dieting can cause you to have a fatty liver—which causes increased blood pressure and higher odds of heart disease. In general, yo-yo dieting makes you feel frustrated and worthless, and the research suggests that weight-cycling is more unhealthy than being overweight. Yo-yo dieting will never give you any satisfaction, so stop the fad diets, stop trying to lose weight, and start making long-term changes that will leave you feeling better about yourself forever.

Create Healthy Habits

Healthy habits are one of the best ways to ensure that you stop binging. If you're able to incorporate some of these habits into your daily life, your body will not feel the same temptation to binge, and your body will thank you for showing it TLC.

Habit 1. Drink more water. You may mistake hunger for needing water, so be sure to keep yourself hydrated. Studies show that people who have water with meals tend to eat less. Furthermore, they feel less hungry at the end of their meals. Carry a water bottle around with you so that you can drink whenever you are thirsty.

Habit 2. Consistently eat meals. Skipping meals is not something that I want you even to consider. I know that diet culture has programmed you into thinking that it's normal to skip meals or replace meals with things like juices, but that's not acceptable. Skipping meals will only make you hungry, and I don't want you to feel hungry. I want you to tend to your body and feel full.

Habit 3. Use meal planning to figure out what you want to eat during the week. Studies have shown that people who use a meal plan tend to have better eating habits. All it takes is for you to take an hour or so each week to decide what you'll want to eat. Also, create a shopping list when you go to the grocery store. Doing so will help prevent you from buying foods you shouldn't.

Habit 4. Feel free to love food. Learn to love cooking it, and don't worry about being around it. Food is not the enemy here. It is good for your body and your mind. Let it do all the things that it should be doing. There's no point in fighting it.

Habit 5. Nourish yourself with things other than food. Focus on your personal relationships, your career, or your spiritual connections to improve your connection between your mind and your body. If you feel nourished in those areas, you will have less need to emotionally eat.

Habit 6. Use your food journal. Write in it every day. This is one of the healthiest habits you can engage in, especially when you're starting your journey to end binging. Remaining vigilant about your eating habits will allow you to better understand your bodily needs and emotional needs when it comes to food.

Habit 7. Honor your cravings. Get in the habit of telling yourself that you can have the foods you crave. Don't get caught up in a restriction mentality. Eat cake at your niece's birthday party without guilt!

Habit 8. Don't let yourself walk away from traditions. You can still have food traditions that remind you of your childhood. Just like you shouldn't deprive yourself of any food, you shouldn't neglect your traditions either because they are part of who you are.

Habit 9. Don't look at food as a punishment or a reward. It's just food. You can enjoy it, but you get to eat it whether you've done well or have failed. You always deserve food, and it's not reflective of how successful you are.

Chapter 5:
Change The Way You Eat…Permanently

A Look at Healthy Meals, Snacks, and Beyond!

Healthy Meals

Healthy meals will include items from all five food groups, so you can mix and match as you please, but here are some options for your consideration.

For all of you who don't eat meat, try a brown rice bowl for your meal. For protein (and grains), you can pair black beans with the rice. For your vegetables, you can add some peppers, tomatoes, and spinach. You can top it all off with some cheese to get your dairy requirement. For dessert, you can have some strawberries with whipped cream to fulfill your fruit requirement.

For you meat-eaters, you can have a healthier version of chicken parmesan. You can have grilled chicken sprinkled with sauce, tomatoes, and a sprinkle of cheese. For your sides, you can have whole grain pasta and steamed broccoli. For dessert, you can have a scoop of ice cream and add a banana to make a banana split. If you don't like any of that, there are plenty of swaps that you can make to include items that you do like. That's the joy of the food groups— you can combine them how you please.

Make an effort to research new dishes and try new food combinations that you've never tried before. Don't let yourself be too safe with what you eat. Some variety will keep you more satisfied than eating the same five things.

Healthy Snacks

There are lots of healthy snacks that can help keep you satiated and feeling good throughout the day. Find snacks that you like and keep your body going.

Nuts are one of the best snacks that you can have because they are very filling and packed with healthy fats. One of my favorite nuts is an almond because almonds taste great, have lots of protein and fiber, and they are easy to bring with me to work or other functions. They are a superfood, making them a great choice for anyone.

Having red bell pepper strips with avocado is another nutritious snack choice. This snack is less portable, but it too is filled with nutrients and healthy fats from the avocado. Moreover, red bell peppers fill you up without being too high in calories.

Apples and a nut butter of your choice are a sweet delicacy. Again, they are filled with fiber, and nut butter (such as almond butter or peanut butter) adds some protein. This snack is both satiating and feels like it's a special treat.

A final snack idea I'll give you is kale chips, which can feed your craving for something crunchy. Being a leafy green vegetable, kale is packed with nutrients and is full of fiber.

Ultimately, be creative with your snacks, but try to find ones that combine a couple of foods to add nutrients that will keep you full between meals.

Be Emotionally Well-Fed

Check-in with how you are feeling throughout your day so that you never starve your emotions of the attention that they need. Even when you are busy, you need to make time to check-in with yourself because if you don't, you'll find yourself being emotionally hungry.

This will ultimately lead to a binge no matter how well you've been eating and physically nourishing yourself.

You cannot have full physical health if you are not mentally healthy. When you're not mentally healthy, all your bodily systems cannot work at peak function. Let yourself feel content with where you are right now so that you can enjoy your food without wanting to overindulge. This is key to defeating binge eating for good.

Get Up and Move – The Benefits of Exercise

Why Exercise?

Exercise may seem like a drag, and it can be arduous work, but it is good for you to get moving. The statistics on physical activity among adults show how inactive people have become. Shockingly, fewer than five percent of adults exercise daily. A hefty eighty percent of adults do not do enough strengthening or aerobic activity. Nearly thirteen percent of people without disabilities aren't active at all during the week. Thus, many people are not experiencing the immense benefits of working out. By adding a little bit of exercise each day, you can transform your life and your relationship to food.

Mood regulation is one significant effect of exercise. Exercise results in your body, releasing endorphins, which make you feel happier. Thus, exercise can help alleviate depression or anxiety. If you're an emotional eater, you know how much your mood can trigger your binging, so get in control of your mood by employing physical activity. To be happy, you must ensure that your body and mind are well taken care of, and exercise can help you do both.

Exercise has an impact on your physical health, of course. It lowers your blood pressure, and it reduces bad cholesterol. Those who exercise also experience better heart health and circulation. They are less likely to get type two diabetes. Exercise is also good for both your bone health and muscle health.

People who exercise sleep better according to research. When you sleep better, you eat better and are less stressed, making sleep directly and indirectly helpful to you—those who exercise sleep for longer and more thoroughly. When you don't get enough sleep, your body's hormones go out of whack. People who get less than seven hours of sleep per night may experience increased ghrelin levels and decreased leptin levels. Ghrelin is the hormone that makes you have an appetite while leptin tells you when you are full. Thus, people who don't get enough sleep not only tend to overeat, but they also tend to choose easy to prepare, high-fat foods that have little nutritional value and do not keep them satiated.

It may not seem like it, but physical activity can make you feel more energized rather than more tired. Those who exercise feel better able to move and accomplish daily life tasks. Moreover, people who are active live longer, and if that's not a good enough reason to get moving, I don't know what is.

Exercising just thirty minutes once a week can improve your binge eating. Doing exercise, no matter how old you are or how inactive, can set you up for a better future, and it's never too late to start, but don't keep waiting to work out. Do it as soon as you finish this book because it will help you make peace with the monster in your mind.

How to Get Moving

You need to get moving, but don't worry about getting moving in the "right" way. There's no wrong way to get moving as long as you are getting your body to be more active. The point is to be active, not to overburden yourself or hurt your body, so don't push yourself past your limits.

Head to the gym. While gyms aren't for everyone, they have a large amount of equipment and classes that you won't be able to find in your house. At a gym, you can get a variety of exercises for one consistent price. Many are open twenty-four seven, making them fairly convenient.

Find a workout buddy. When I started exercising, I was shy about going to the gym, so I asked my best friend if she would be interested in heading to the gym with me. We both wanted to get more active, so it worked out well for both of us. Having someone to get active with makes the experience markedly more enjoyable, and you can keep each other accountable so that you don't slack off.

Take an exercise class. Lots of gyms and studios have fun workout classes led by instructors. Yoga, pilates, Zumba, ballet barre, and other work out programs can get your blood pumping while still being fun. Many include dance elements and great music!

Go outdoors. Walking, hiking or biking are all some good options for both getting active and enjoying the great outdoors. If you have a pool in your yard or a local outdoor pool, swimming is a fantastic low-impact option for people looking to strengthen their bodies. Being outside feels meditative and less rigid than going to the gym for many people.

Workout at home. Whether you get equipment, use recorded workout programs, play fitness games, or even just walk up and down your steps, you can get an extensive workout at home.

Journal about your progress. Your fitness goals and progress reports have a place in your journal. Write down how much you move and what kind of exercises you do. Try to build up and improve your skillsets as you go. Write down things you want to be able to do with your body in the future and plan to work towards those goals.

Search the internet for workouts. There's plenty of workouts at the touch of your fingers, so don't be afraid to scour the internet for different programs that might meet your skills and fitness needs.

Get a personal trainer. If you're feeling a bit lost, it may help to have a personal trainer who can guide you about proper workout procedures and make sure that you don't hurt yourself by using certain equipment the wrong way.

Whatever it is that you do, make sure that you enjoy it. Working out won't always be pleasant, but it needs to make you feel satisfied and healthy.

With a Little Help From My Friends

You should get your friends involved in your process to end binge eating. Binge eating is such a solitary experience that working through it alone feels overwhelming. When my life was shrouded in secrecy, and even the closest people to me didn't realize what I was going through, I felt so depressed, and I wondered if I'd ever be motivated to get better.

Breakthrough your shame and tell friends what has been going on with you because sharing this awful experience will lift a weight from your shoulders, and your friendship will be better once you are honest. You'll be more vulnerable and share deep, important parts of yourself that you felt you needed to hide in the past.

Eat with friends. When I eat with friends, I'm distracted from the food in front of me, and while you may still feel urges to binge, it's much easier to stay on track when you're not eating alone. Plan to have as many meals as you can with other people. It may feel mortifying at first, or you may feel silly asking friends or loved ones to eat meals with you, but it does help.

Don't let your pride stand in the way of letting your friends do what they can to help you. Your loved ones want you to be happy and healthy, and their offers of help shouldn't be taken defensively. Be sure to tell them when they've stepped too far, but allow them to help when they can because you need their support.

Give your friends boundaries. Accepting help is wonderful, but we all have certain boundaries that we need to maintain, or else relationships start to crumble and feel toxic. Let them know things that trigger you and will only make you worse. Put your recovery first!

Spend more time with your friends. Being social is important to human well-being. Accordingly, the simple act of spending more time with people who you love can empower you and make you feel more comfortable in your own skin. When you spend time with your friends, focus on your relationships with those people rather than your relationship with food. Your friends deserve your attention too, so be there for them as much as they are there for you. Don't be scared to try new things with the people you love. Expand your boundaries and create new memories with your friends.

Ask your friends to hold you accountable, and keep them updated on your progress. Share the obstacles along with the successes. Let them know how you've been doing so that they can push you to continue to make progress. Never revert to being ashamed. Find at least one person who will listen to your struggles and celebrate your victories. You have a rocky path ahead of you, and sometimes, you'll fall, but you'll get to your destination with friends who are willing to pull you up.

Cut out any toxic friends. People who make you feel bad about yourself should have no place in your life. Losing friends is hard, and walking away from friendships takes courage, but sometimes doing so is vital. If people cannot accept you as you are, then they are not worth keeping around because they'll only cause you heartache.

Don't be afraid to ask for advice or your friend's open ear. If you need to talk, don't keep what you have to say bottled up. Writing your feelings down is helpful, but confessing them to a waiting ear can be even more cathartic. Be bold and talk about your emotions so that your feelings cannot get the best of you. Your friends might even give you some new insight that you never considered before, speeding up your recovery process substantially.

Value yourself as your friends value you. I used to always think my friends were too great to truly like someone like me. I figured that it was a fluke that they chose to hang out with me when I wasn't anyone special or cool, but the thing is that my friends *did* think that I was special and cool. They saw qualities about me that I couldn't see. Try to look at yourself from that perspective and realize that the negativity you have about yourself is not how other people look at you.

Your friends are some of the most important people in your life. They may even be like family to you. You've been through a lot together, I'm sure, and you can get through binge eating too. This is not a battle you have to fight alone. You have allies, and it's time to turn to them and let them into this part of your life.

Never Give Up, Never Surrender

Why You Should Persist

You need to persist through your recovery process even if it seems hard because recovering from your binge eating is going to change your entire future. You have two options. You can either continue your life as it is, or you can change. Persist past all the pain. Persist past all the cravings. Persist past all the slipups. Move past all the hardship, and you'll finally be free from binging your life away. Your future is in your hands, and the beautiful thing is that you're the one who defines what happens next. There's so much that you can't predict in your future, but no matter who you are, you can craft a future worth living.

How to Get Through Hardship

Believe in yourself. This is the most important thing that you can do. Don't doubt your ability to get through this. If you say that you will never stop binging, you will never stop binging. That's the bottom line. You become your inner dialogue, so starting telling yourself that you will succeed. Write it on sticky notes and repeat it to yourself each time you wake up, and each time you go to bed. Repeat after me, "I will succeed. I will be free from binge eating. I will be fully me, and I will not let my disorder control who I will be."

Know that obstacles aren't the death of progress. If you've abstained from binging for a week and then find yourself binging again, you don't have to keep binging. A slip up doesn't mean that you've failed at recovery. I cannot tell you how many times I slipped up and went back to binging. I'd go weeks or months without it, and then I'd find myself back to doing it again, but I didn't give up. I used those mistakes to make myself even more determined to get better. Be stubborn, and don't let obstacles define what will become of you.

Remember that as long as you are trying to get better then you *are* getting better. You are better than you were when you weren't trying to cure your disorder. You've already made substantial progress coming this far. The hardest part is admitting to yourself that you have a problem. All that's left is to fight for recovery and always keep your end goals in sight. Never forget why you are trying to get better. You're trying to save yourself from the misery of binging. You're doing your best, and you will find peace soon. Just hold on a little longer.

Don't forget that you're through the worst of your binging. If you're reading this book, you don't have to let your binge eating get worse. Your worst day can already be over, and from here, it will be uphill. Recovery is like a mountain range. You have ups and downs that you have to travel across, but you'll get better at managing the terrain, and you'll learn how to get yourself through the lows so that when the highs come, you can enjoy your breathtaking surroundings. As long as you are practicing recovery, you can never be kicked down forever, so get up on your feet, and let's go!

Living With the Long-Term Results

Changes That Last

If you want long-term results, you have to make changes that will last. Don't look at these changes as something you can stop once you finally stop binge eating. You have to continue these practices for the rest of your life. They will become more instinctual, but you'll never be able to go on a diet again because going on a diet would bring you right back where you started. You can't make losing weight your main purpose, either. If it happens, it happens, but it may not. Make peace with the fact that the number on the scale might not change (but your body certainly will when you stop binging).

Tell yourself that you can make lasting change. Self-doubt is only going to create a self-fulfilling prophecy. Believe in this process and give it your all. Adjust my recommendations to your specific needs, but let yourself give these steps and tools a valiant try because I guarantee that you won't be worse off for them.

Keep the person you want to be in mind, and know that there are lots of success stories. You can be that person who you're dreaming of being. It may take a lot of work to get there, but there is hope for you. Anyone who sets their mind to it can end the binge-restrict cycle.

How to Stick to a Plan

Sticking to a plan is hard for many people, but fear not, there are steps that you can take to ensure that you don't wander from your aspirations.

Write your plan down. Hopefully, you've already done this in the planning portion of the book. Mental health experts generally use the acronym S.M.A.R.T. to dictate what goals should look like: specific, measurable, achievable, realistic, and timely. Keep these terms in mind as you're trying to keep to your plan. Post sticky notes around your house to easily remember what you are working towards. The more you are exposed to your goals, the better your results will be. Don't just write them down, though, repeat your goals out loud because doing so will help your brain absorb your aspirations even more.

Don't do too much at once. Focus on one behavior that you need to change, and then once you accomplish that, work on others. Taking on too many behaviors at once will only overwhelm you. It's better to take your time to stop your binge eating than to rush through, so work on one issue at once and add more as you feel comfortable doing so.

Make manageable deadlines that make up smaller goals and build to your larger goal. Deadlines are good because they are quantifiable, but be careful not to make them too rigid. Furthermore, don't make your only deadlines long-term. Have milestones leading up to the longer-term deadlines. You should also note that deadlines aren't the end-all and be-all of success. If you miss a deadline, you can still succeed. Look at the deadlines as an ETA rather than as a time you need to be there. By doing this, you can take some of the pressure off, which will make it easier to reach your goals. You will progress at your own pace, but you can push yourself to move at your quickest rate.

Have a non-food related prize for when you reach your goals. This prize can be anything that you want. Maybe you want to buy new clothes, or maybe you want to buy your family a dog. Whatever it is that you want, reward yourself along the way. While you won't get instant gratification, you can still be gratified at various points in the process.

Hold yourself accountable for when you don't reach your goals. Don't look at mishaps as failures. Instead, see them as opportunities to do better. Whenever you miss your goal, it's a chance to learn and know what to do differently next time.

Conclusion

As our time together comes to a close, I want to review all the progress you've made during this book, and the lessons you've learned because believe it or not, the strides you've made are significant. The information you've read here will serve you for the rest of your life. I hope you can apply these lessons to yourself and find the freedom that you deserve. Progress may be slow, but it will come.

I've been free of binge eating for years, but it also took me years to get to this point, and even now, there are still days when I struggle. Food does not run my life. I am free, and I want more than anything for you to be free as well because no one deserves to live with the binge monster inside of them. Binge eating is a dark, lonely disorder, but it's not incurable.

You've gone to the root of your binge eating, and examined the personal and cultural aspects that may influence your binge eating. If you didn't know, you learned the difference between mere overeating and binge eating. You learned how prevalent food issues are in our culture and how these issues are influenced by societal, environmental, and biological factors. Hopefully, you realized that you are far from alone in your binge eating. Too often, binge eating is normalized or made into a joke on sitcoms, but it is a real issue that devastates lives and makes it hard for people to engage in regular activities, particularly ones that are related to food. Continue to dig into why you started binge eating and under what conditions you do it because these answers will guide you as you make recovery permanent.

You've discovered the joy of eating slowly and the importance of slowing down your rapid thoughts by journaling. You need to appreciate your food rather than stuffing it into your face as fast as possible. Slow eating allows you to be more mindful and keeps your hunger cue engaged, so you don't fill yourself past your limit. You've learned to resist the urge of instant gratification and to realize that you must wait for progress because it takes months or even years to improve your binge eating. Make incremental goals that power you through each day and motivate you to continue striving for your best. To stay mindful of your eating habits and your goals, you can use a food journal to track what you're eating and how you feel when you're eating it, among other aspirations such as exercise goals or food ideas. You've learned to listen to your hunger, both emotional and physical, which will benefit you in the rest of this process.

You've seen the power of nutrition and the types of foods that you should be eating to make sure your body feels nourished and doesn't want to binge. The urge to binge often biologically stems from being deprived. The Minnesota Starvation Experiment shows that people become obsessed with food even when only moderately deprived, leading to binging. Furthermore, dividing foods into the categories of good and bad can be equally dangerous because doing so creates a similar restriction mindest. It makes you feel deprived. Your body fears that it is going to starve, so it eats as much as it can. While foods aren't good or bad, you need to pay attention to what you are eating because certain foods are more satiating than others, and if you want your body to be satisfied, you need to get all your nutrients. Be sure to include all five food groups as well as the three main macronutrients and the micronutrients, which include vitamins and minerals, in your diet.

You've created a strategy to curb overeating and take back your body. Find ways to manage your stress. Don't let your emotions decide what you're going to eat. Take the power of your body back. Include more fiber and protein in your diet because they are good for digestion and satiation. Plus, they have a myriad of other health benefits that will boost your energy. Learn to plan for your future, including your goals and meals, and practice swapping emotional eating for healthier options that will give you the energy to get up and live your life.

You've learned how to manage your feelings and personal life in ways that aren't overeating; these skills will help you create long-term change and allow you to be free for the rest of your life. Be creative when including healthy meals, snacks, and emotional energy into your diet. Have fun trying new things and exploring healthy dishes. Another great way to manage your binge eating recovery is to get up and move. Incorporate more exercise into your life and have fun doing it. Further, don't handle your struggles alone. Invite friends into your personal life and allow them to help you get better. Don't let yourself give up on your progress. Believe in yourself so that you can live with the long-term results and never go back to how you were before. There's no time for turning back. Reach out for your future and take it.

In all these lessons, I have taught you why you are binge eating and how you can put an end to it without having to torture yourself with dieting or eating foods that you hate. I've shown that you can successfully eliminate binging while still being the person you've always been. My goal was never to change who you are but to allow that person to exist again after being suffocated by binge eating for so long because that person deserves to feel fully alive.

I appreciate you reaching the end of *Stop Binge Eating 101*, and I sincerely hope that it gave you the tools and information that you need to end your battle with binge eating forever.

What I need you to do now is to put this plan into action and finally free yourself from binge eating. There's no looking back. Don't wait until tomorrow to do it. Change your life right now, and if you don't take anything else away from this book, I want you to know that there's nothing to be ashamed of if you are a binge eater. Your dignity and worth as a person are not changed based on what you eat, and I hope you can love yourself and embrace the unique person who you are. Binging or not, you're still the same amazing person you have always been!